A Family Caregiver Speaks Up

Also by Suzanne Geffen Mintz

The Resourceful Caregiver:
Helping Family Caregivers Help Themselves

Love, Honor, & Value: A Family Caregiver Speaks Out about the
Choices & Challenges of Caregiving (Capital, 2002)

A Family Caregiver Speaks Up

"It Doesn't Have to Be This Hard"

Suzanne Geffen Mintz
President, Co-Founder
National Family Caregivers Association

CAPITAL CARES SERIES

CAPITAL
BOOKS, INC.
Sterling, Virginia

Capital Books, Inc.
P.O. Box 605
Herndon, Virginia 20172-0605

ISBN 13: 978-1-933102-46-7

Library of Congress Cataloging-in-Publication Data

Mintz, Suzanne.
 A Family caregiver speaks up : it doesn't have to be this hard / Suzanne Geffen Mintz.
     p. cm. — (Capital cares series)
Rev. ed. of: Love, honor & value. 2002.
Includes bibliographical references.
ISBN 978-1-933102-46-7 (alk. paper)
1. Caregivers. I. Mintz, Suzanne Love, honor & value. II. Title. III. Series.

RA645.35.M54 2007
649.8—dc22

          2007034238

Printed in the United States of America on acid-free paper that meets the American National Standards Institute Z39-48 Standard.

First Edition

10 9 8 7 6 5 4 3 2 1

For Steven and Cindy, always,
and in memory of Dana Reeve

∾ *Contents* ∾

∾ *Foreword* ∾

I first met Suzanne Mintz at a conference on caregiving and long-term care. I'd heard that she was a passionate caregiver, with a good grasp of the issues and a vision of how caregiving families should be treated. After meeting her I knew why. Bound by the zeal that only a person with first-hand experience as a caregiver can bring, Suzanne has become an advocate extraordinaire for caregiving families. Putting in words the thoughts and feelings of millions of family caregivers, she gives a voice to the voiceless and minimizes the frustration that so often comes to those who provide care for a chronically ill, disabled, or aged loved one.

Launching a national organization, the National Family Caregivers Association (NFCA), was the logical step when she and long-time friend Cindy Fowler realized that family caregiving is a lifespan issue that brings similar concerns and problems regardless of relationship or a loved one's diagnosis. Today NFCA is one of the largest and most influential organizations for family caregivers in the country, providing information and education, support and validation, and public awareness and advocacy, all in an effort to make life better for family caregivers and their loved ones. And now this book that provides both personal accounts—hers and many others—combined with practical advice and a call to action for family caregivers, is here to make sure caregivers' voices are heard, and their difficulties are known to other family members and friends, within their local communities, and in the halls of county, state, and national government.

Family Caregiver Alliance (FCA), the San Francisco-based organization I am proud to direct, was created out of similar circumstances. Individual family caregivers Anne Bashkiroff and Suzanne Harris were willing to talk about their private experiences in public so others would not have to face the isolation, confusion, and lack of support from the medical community that were created by their role as primary providers of care for their loved ones with Alzheimer's. Their efforts and those of a few other caregiver advocates and interested professionals gave birth to what is now a thirty-year-old organization known nationally for its ability to provide policy makers, program developers, and researchers with the information they need to further their work in assisting family caregivers.

It's hard to believe that from such humble beginnings, from the fire of a few, so much can happen. And yet that is the way of progress and change, and NFCA and FCA have proved that a few committed people really can make a difference. Many other grassroots organizations can trace their history back to a few advocates who defined a dream and enlisted the support of others to make it come true. They told their stories in an effort to right the wrongs they saw and experienced on a daily level, and in the process heightened the awareness and brought forth the hidden energy of others. They planted the seeds of a movement they may never have imagined possible.

Caregiving families face innumerable challenges on a daily basis. Changes in the care a loved one needs creates a whole new reality for the caregiver. Some family caregivers learn to anticipate. Others can't and are always thrown into crises. Family and friends drift away after the acute stage of an illness is over because they are uncomfortable facing the reality of growing disability or unusual behaviors. Simultaneous work and care responsibilities squeeze all personal time from the calendar of a caregiver, and denying their own health problems in the face of daily caregiving demands unfortunately is commonplace—all of these are part of the reality of being a family caregiver, and they all come to life in this book through the quotes of caregivers from across the country.

> *At each step we have tried to anticipate the next problem Dad would be facing. . . . This forward thinking has helped us not have to scramble and has helped us be mentally prepared as changes occurred.*
>
> —Indiana

> *A lot of people don't want to be around someone who is sick. Some friends may never call or stop by again.*
>
> —California

> *. . . have nurses during the day to care for Kaylee so I can work and I have nurses at night so I can sleep. . . . I have* NO *time to care for myself.*
>
> —Maryland

> *After three months I had lost twenty pounds, had terrible bags under my eyes, and looked like a zombie. The doctor threatened to hospitalize me because I was suffering from exhaustion.*
>
> —New Jersey

All these conditions pose problems for family caregivers and, although they are lived out in individual lives, they demand service solutions that are comprehensive in their approach, solutions that acknowledge all caregivers' rights to information, sources of support, recognition of their own physical and mental health issues, and legal and financial considerations.

Family caregivers are the "care coordinators" of their family. Long-term care is not measured in months or by individual crises, but rather by years and maintenance of loved ones' functions. Family caregivers are the historians and managers of their loved one's medical, social, financial, and cultural lives. Seen in this light, it is clear that the issues involved in supporting family caregivers are complex. They are personal. They are familial, and yes, they are societal too. And yet, so many family caregivers are not aware that all of these issues are swirling around them and that more than 50 million other Americans, just like them, are providing some level of care to a loved one in need. The isolation that so often accompanies caregiving deprives them of even the slim support of knowing they are not alone.

A Family Caregiver Speaks Up explores what this means in the everyday lives of family caregivers, and what each of us might be able to do to meet our individual challenges. It discusses why caregiving is different today than it was in the past and suggests what society ought to do to integrate family caregiving into the fabric of our healthcare system. It honors the work of family caregivers by explaining how caregivers are actually members of their loved one's healthcare team, and how much knowledge of their loved one's condition they bring to the table.

By sharing the story of her personal journey combined with a call to action, Suzanne has made a difference in the lives of the family caregivers who have heard her speak or read her articles. Now with the publication of this book, so many more people will have the chance to learn, to feel, to be inspired, and in some cases to follow her lead.

Thanks, Suzanne, for coming forward with your story so others may not have to face the isolation, confusion, and lack of support so common with families caring for their loved ones, and thank you for starting the National Family Caregivers Association so that caregivers all across the country, regardless of their circumstances, can know there is a better way and that there are many of us around the country working to make a vision of a better world for caregiving families come true.

Kathleen A. Kelly
Executive Director
Family Caregiver Alliance

～ *Acknowledgments* ～

It has been five years since the first edition of this book was published, and I remain so very grateful to all of those who helped bring it into being.

Much has happened in this five-year period. I have learned and grown as a person and NFCA has grown as an organization. I have been most fortunate to have great advisers along the way who made that growth possible, key among them: Christal Willingham, Deborah Halpern, Brooks Kenny, and Stephe McMahon. Members of NFCA's Caregiver Community Action Network (CCAN), led by board member Linda Jones, have been a wonderful help, as have the other members of the NFCA board who continue to teach me to think in new ways.

The most extensive changes have been made to chapter three—"It Doesn't Have to Be This Hard." I am very grateful to Anne Montgomery and Piper Su for reading this chapter and providing me with their comments. NFCA's public policy team at the law firm of Patton Boggs and Jill Kagan of the National Respite Coalition have been especially helpful in expanding my understanding of the legislative process, and I am grateful to Kathleen Hughes of Capital Books for believing in the value of this second edition. A special thank you to Jane Cortez and Joanne Cruz for their help in updating statistics for this new edition.

A personal thank you to Cindy, without whom all of this wouldn't have been possible, for being such a true friend.

And to Steven, who watches out for me, and whom I love dearly and always will.

All proceeds due the author
from the sale of
A Family Caregiver Speaks Up
are being donated to the
National Family Caregivers Association.
NFCA is a 501(c)3 Organization.
Tax ID # is 52 - 1780405

∾ Introduction ∾
to the Second Edition

The advice and ideas I shared in the first edition of this book about how to make your caregiving life somewhat easier continue to ring true to me, but five years is a long time and much has happened since 2002 in the larger environment that impacts the lives of all caregiving families, including my own, and that is why I have decided to update and revise portions of this book.

If you read the first edition, you will already have noticed that the title of this edition has changed from *Love, Honor, & Value: A Family Caregiver Speaks Out about the Choices and Challenges of Caregiving* to *A Family Caregiver Speaks Up: "It Doesn't Have to Be This Hard."*

The title's emphasis has shifted from the emotions and day-to-day practical details of life as a family caregiver, to my belief that being a family caregiver is much harder than it needs to be, and that there are things that we all can do to change that. Much of the book still focuses on the emotions and day-to-day issues that impact caregiving families; indeed how could it not? They are the reality of our lives. And although some of the chapter headings have been altered slightly, to align with updated wording of NFCA's core principles, the copy within them has only changed when it needed to be updated. These core principles are: believe in yourself; protect your health; reach out for help; speak up for your rights. Time has shown that taking these messages to heart enables family caregivers to be more proactive, feel more confident and empowered, and thereby have more control over their lives. All these topics are discussed in the book, as they were in the first edition, but "It Doesn't Have to Be This Hard" (formerly "Beyond You and Me") appears near the beginning of the book now to emphasize my message that there is a real need for systemic change to improve the quality of life for caregiving families.

In the introduction to the first edition I referred to a definition of family caregivers I thought was the best I had ever heard. I have yet to find a better one, and therefore I am including it here again as the foundation of our journey together through the pages of this book.

> *Marjorie is a family caregiver, a person who provides essential, unpaid assistance to a relative or friend who is ill, elderly, or disabled. The two parts of the term are equally important. "Family" denotes a special personal relationship with the care recipient; one based on birth, adoption, marriage, or declared commitment. "Caregiver" is the job description, which may include providing personal care, carrying out medical procedures, managing a household, and interacting with the formal healthcare and social service systems on another's behalf. Caregivers are more than the sum of their responsibilities; they are real people with complex and often conflicted responses to the situations they face.*

This description of the term *family caregiver* was written by Carol Levine, in *Always on Call: When Illness Turns Families into Caregivers*. Carol is the director of the Families and Health Care Project at the United Hospital Fund of New York. The description reflects her professional knowledge of the issues of family caregiving and also her very personal understanding of what it means to be a family caregiver. She cared for her husband, who was severely injured in an automobile accident more than seventeen years ago, until his death this past December.

Carol's distinction between the word *family* as the definer of a caring relationship and the word *caregiver* as the description of a job is an important one. Putting the two together as a single term is what distinguishes you and me from others who provide care, such as doctors, nurses, homecare aides, and members of the clergy, none of whom fit the description above, largely because the care they provide stems from the careers they have chosen to pursue. Nonetheless these professionals, and especially the paraprofessionals, think of themselves as caregivers and so does the wider world.

This book continues to be about family caregivers not professional ones. It uses the term *family caregiver* in the broadest sense possible and it uses the terms *family caregiver* and *caregiver* interchangeably. It was written primarily for current family caregivers, but I hope it will also find a ready audience among policy makers, members of the health and social services communities, and those in line to become family caregivers.

It was difficult for me to define the exact nature of the first edition of my book, and it still is. It isn't a caregiver's memoir, although it certainly contains personal information about my own caregiving experience. It puts forth a philosophy of family caregiver self-advocacy and suggests ways to live your life well as a family caregiver, but it in no way claims that this is the only way to do that. It's not a workbook, although it does ask questions and does provide suggestions for activities. It is not a collection of other caregivers' thoughts, feelings, and ideas, although these are definitely sprinkled throughout the book, and despite the added emphasis on the connection between public policy and the daily lives of caregiving families in this edition, it is not a treatise. I invite you to read it and decide for yourself.

In 2002 the book was written based on the information, and hopefully wisdom, I had gained from my own ongoing caregiving journey, and the knowledge, empathy, and education I gained since co-founding NFCA in 1993. This second edition builds on that knowledge and experience, both personal and professional, and I hope that reading this new edition will provide you with some "ah-ha" moments that help make a positive difference in your life, your loved one's life, and the lives of at least some of the more than 50 million other family caregivers in America who also struggle each day to find some equilibrium in their lives.

Suzanne Mintz
Kensington, MD
May 2007

~ CHAPTER 1 ~

In Sickness and in Health

It all began on a Sunday afternoon in the fall of 1974 when my husband, Steven, began feeling a tingling sensation in both legs. He tried shaking them, the way you do when they've "fallen sleep." But that didn't make the tingling sensation go away. It persisted during the rest of the day and throughout the night. So in the morning, Steven called our internist and friend, Dr. Hal Mirsky, in the hope of getting an appointment later that day. But Hal advised otherwise. "I think you should see a neurologist rather than me," he said. "I'll give you a referral." That's how we met Dr. Richard Edelson. After hearing Steven's symptoms and doing a number of non-invasive tests in his office, Dr. Edelson said that Steven should enter George Washington University Hospital right away. More tests were necessary. It was obvious that something was definitely wrong, and both Steven and I started to get scared.

He was in the hospital for four or five days. It's hard to remember exactly. Time didn't seem to be following its regular steady pattern. Some days a second felt like an hour, and on other days hours flew by like seconds as I tried to keep up with the normal routine of life and spend as much time at the hospital with Steven as was possible.

Some of the tests didn't seem like tests at all. The doctor would bang Steven's knees with a triangular shaped hammer

1

to see how quickly they jutted forward. He asked him lots of questions. "Do you ever recall not being able to get one of your legs to respond in the normal way, either while you were walking or running? Do you ever recall stubbing your toe while climbing stairs? Any problems seeing? Any difficulty picking up things with your hands? Do you get overly fatigued in the heat?" The questions horrified me, one of Steven's answers even more. He acknowledged having a problem with his right leg from time to time. That explained, to me at least, why he always had an excuse for not wanting to play basketball with the other men in our garden-apartment complex. An athlete and sports lover, he wasn't willing to join the game if he couldn't perform at the level he was used to. There was some good news coupled with the bad. The problem, whatever it was, seemed to be localized. Symptoms had never appeared anywhere other than his right leg.

Dr. Edelson ordered a number of tests that, in themselves, were frightening. For one of them, a mylogram, Steven was fastened to a table and turned upside down. A dye was injected into his spinal column, so that the doctors could watch the dye on a monitor as it flowed from the base of his spinal column all the way up into his neck. They wanted to see if there were any blockages along the column that might explain the tingling. The test was done while Steven was wide-awake because it was vital that he be conscious and not move even a fraction of an inch so that the dye wouldn't flow further than intended. He still recalls the anxiety and fear as he watched the dye flow ever closer to his brain and the point of danger, and the sigh of relief he let out when the test was finally over.

He was warned that another test would give him significant headaches. It involved inserting a needle into his spinal column and drawing out fluid. The fluid would then be tested to measure the level of various proteins, especially gamma globulin. Although it wouldn't prove anything conclusively, we were told, given the technology of the time, that it was our best shot at finding out what was wrong. He should expect the headaches to last about two weeks, until his body had time to regenerate the lost spinal fluid and restore its balance. Although the test was dangerous, as you can imagine removing spinal fluid has to be done very, very carefully, we decided Steven should go ahead with it. We wanted to know what was happening to his body and why.

Some images from that time are still very vivid for me. I recall the evenings when Steven was in the hospital. After our daughter, Darryn, all of five years old, had been put to bed, and I finished my chores and homework (I was in graduate school at the time), I'd get into bed myself, emotionally and physically weary, and I would cry. Violent sobs escaped from my mouth, and I tried to muffle them with my hand, afraid that Darryn might wake and want to know why I was crying. I'd lay there, arms crossed in front of my chest squeezing my upper arms, trying without much success to feel that I was being held and comforted. "Perhaps he'll need an operation, perhaps he'll need an operation, perhaps he'll need an operation," I said silently to myself, seeing brain surgery not as something to fear but rather the potential answer to my prayers. I prayed to God, whom I never before believed was a direct interventionist in our individual lives, but whom, during those nights, I fervently wished was. I prayed that Steven would be well. I wanted to know what was happening to his body. I wanted an answer. I wanted whatever was wrong to be made right. Eventually I would fall asleep and wake in the morning as tired as I had been when I went to bed.

There are some memories from that time that are more than vivid. They are imprinted on my heart forever. The moment I heard Steven's diagnosis is one of them. The details are still crystal clear, even though it happened more than thirty years ago.

It was a crisp, sunny day in October, I had gone to the hospital and as I was getting off the elevator the attending physician on duty came over to me. "I was hoping I would see you," he said, guiding me to the waiting area, a rather public and very uninviting space furnished with cheap, plastic, molded chairs that were lined up in rows facing each other.

"Your husband has multiple sclerosis," he continued without emotion. "MS is a degenerative and incurable neurological disease. I'm sorry." An image from childhood flashed through my mind, the image of a neighbor who had MS. I would see her, on sunny days, sitting on her front porch in a wheelchair as I walked up the street with the jaunty step of a preteen on the way to play with a friend. I don't recall if I ever said hello. I hope I did. I now envisioned Steven in a wheelchair wrapped up in a blanket the way Mrs. Schmirer always was, waiting for someone to bring her a glass of water with a straw, or wheel her back into the house. It was so terrifying it took my breath away. I was twenty-eight years old when Steven was diagnosed with MS. He was thirty-one. From that moment on, our lives and Darryn's were irrevocably changed.

Steven had a very different reaction to the news. He didn't know anything about MS. He'd never seen anyone with it. No images popped into his head. The words didn't create the same sense of fear and dread in him that they immediately did in me. The doctor had told him the same things he had told me and so he was scared about what could happen—who wouldn't be—but no specific images, no memories of real people haunted him.

Not long after he was diagnosed I heard that people with multiple sclerosis have a high divorce rate. Whether it is true or not I don't really know. I never wanted to actually find out for fear that it would happen to us. It wouldn't surprise me though. The vagaries of the disease, its often on-again-off-again nature, its degenerative path, and the fact that it usually attacks just when a person is spreading his or her adult wings, all conspire to eat away at the tender core of a marriage. MS has no specific prognosis, no timetable, no cure. If it's mild, symptoms may recede or go away entirely for long periods of time. If it's more virulent, the damage accumulates in very visible ways. Today there are drugs that help slow the progress of the disease, but in 1974 there wasn't anything of the sort available. Flair ups could be treated, but the disease would take its own willful course. That's one of the things that makes it so devastating. There's nothing about MS you can hang your hat on, nothing that points the way to a specific plan of action. You know it's there. The words have been uttered. It is now part of your medical history. Like an uninvited guest that has made himself at home, it has somehow become a permanent part of your family.

When Steven came home from the hospital, the tingles had stopped, and nothing seemed different about him. He'd stub a toe on a step now and then, unable to move his foot in quite the right way to easily climb from riser to riser, but that was all. Why make anyone worry, we thought, deciding not to tell our parents, all four of whom lived in Florida, or even our closest friends that we saw all the time and thought of as family. But I desperately needed to feel I wasn't on my own in dealing with the knowledge of Steven's diagnosis and my fears about our future. And so we took Steven's sister and brother-in-law into our confidence. It helped a little, but the fact that they too lived far away meant I still didn't have a shoulder to cry on in the literal sense.

Outwardly, the pattern of our lives didn't change. Darryn entered first grade. I completed my master's degree and got a part-time job with a design firm—my first paid employment since she was born, and Steven continued to work as an economist for the federal government.

Everything seemed normal, but nothing was. Our sensitivities were so heightened that the simplest questions—"how was your day?"—took on a new significance. The response, "it was tiring," conjured up an invalid's lifestyle. I was apprehensive, unsure of what might happen from day to day, unsure of every conversation, unsure of being too solicitous or of not showing enough concern. Steven's health became a major topic of conversation. It consumed our attention and stifled me, but I couldn't admit it. I couldn't say, "Let's not talk about how you feel all of the time. Let's try and live as normal a life as possible."

Steven, never one to share much about his inner feelings, shared even less of them then. I didn't know whether he felt the same about the turn our conversations had taken. I didn't know what he needed to quiet his personal fear of the unknown, but I later learned neither did he. We were hurting very badly, grieving the loss of what we thought life should and would be like. Neither one of us had any immediate answers. We were both just trying, in our different ways, to survive emotionally.

On top of the confusion and pain that Steven's diagnosis brought into our lives, another catastrophic event occurred nine months later. This one happened to me, to my body. I was raped. At home. In my own bed. Steven was away on a business trip. Darryn was asleep in the next room and a man broke into our apartment. He woke me out of a deep sleep, pulled the blanket over my head, and said, "If you don't stay quiet and keep your eyes covered, I'll bruise you." Once I became fully conscious and realized what was happening, my greatest fear was that Darryn would wake up and walk into my bedroom. "What might happen then? What would he do to her?" I lay there as he commanded, not moving a muscle, and when he got what he came for, he left as silently as he had come. It happened relatively quickly and without any violence whatsoever. It would have been easy to think I had imagined it, but I knew I hadn't, and so with the day slowly dawning outside my window, I called 911.

The police officers who came in response to my call, a man and a woman, were great. They treated me with respect and compassion. They said I'd have to go to the hospital and have an internal examination to corroborate my story. For the second time in the space of only a few hours I was to have a stranger explore the most intimate part of my body. A neighbor took Darryn and off I went in the police car. Once at the hospital I remember sitting on the examination table, waiting and waiting and waiting for the doctor to appear. The policewoman stayed with me the whole time. I was so grateful. A social worker came in and gave me her card. "Call me," she said. "I think it will be good for you to talk about this." Finally the doctor came, unceremoniously examined me and said that yes, I had definitely been raped. Then he left and I was free to go home. I had no physical wounds that needed to heal, so there were no outward physical reminders of my ordeal, but for months I heard the rapist's voice in my ears, and I wonder to this very day if the emotional wounds he left behind have fully healed, or if they ever will.

The police never did find out who the rapist was, or how he got into our apartment. The balcony faced dark woods, and they thought he might have climbed up the railing to our third floor apartment and entered through the sliding glass doors. We also never found out if it was a random act or if I was the intended victim. With all that uncertainty neither Steven nor I felt safe in the apartment, and for Steven, it was a constant reminder that he hadn't been home that night, even though he knew that if he had the outcome might have been worse than it was.

The bad memories and unanswered questions prompted us to buy our first house, a happy event brought about by unhappy circumstances. We bought a ranch-style house, just in case Steven wouldn't be able to climb stairs one day. The change of scene was helpful, but in the months and years that followed Steven and I were overwhelmed with what had happened to each of our bodies and to our collective lives.

We needed to come to terms with the two great traumas we had suffered, and we didn't know how. We each needed to grieve, but didn't understand why, or know that grieving is a very personal act that all of us need to experience in our own way, according to our inner workings. Little did we know that our grieving styles and coping mechanisms were completely opposite each other. Little did we know that our inability to share what we were each really thinking and feeling and needing would soon have a disastrous effect on our relationship.

Steven's natural inclination is to turn inward for strength. I need to reach out for support. It never occurred to us that these differences would cause us to end up waging an emotional war against each other, a war that would lead to a ten-month separation, followed by an eighteen-month truce and another separation, this one lasting two full years, before we finally realized just how different we were emotionally. It was a profound awakening when we came to understand that neither Steven's way of coping nor mine was better, but rather that their differences needed to be recognized and respected if we were to live comfortably together under one roof again.

Darryn lived with me during the two years we were apart, but she saw Steven every weekend and helped him with the groceries. We were constantly concerned about her reaction to Steven's increasing disability and our separation. Her best friend's dad was disabled and her parents divorced so the girls became an emotional lifeline for each other and developed a very deep bond that continues to this day. Darryn constantly assured me that she was okay, and I had no reason not to take her at her word, but I was also glad that she had Shannon to talk to during those difficult times.

Like most couples, Steven and I had married "for better or for worse, in sickness and in health." But nobody who marries at twenty-one, as I did, or at twenty-three as Steven did, thinks that means anything more serious than the common cold. No young couple expects tragedy to invade their lives.

I think the reason we were able to heal our marriage despite the many serious injuries it had received is that underneath it all we really are quite good for each other. Darryn said it best, when we asked her if she had been concerned that we might actually get divorced. "No," she responded. "I knew you guys loved each other." So after years of turmoil and heartache, we got together again, this time truly for better or for worse, but the hardest part was still ahead.

Steven has the slow, continually degenerating variety of MS, technically called *primary progressive*. It is the least common of the three types. Like a leaky faucet that only attracts attention after water starts to visibly collect in the basin, primary progressive MS drips into your life. By 1979, five years after his diagnosis, Steven's basin was filling up. His gait was uneven, his balance a bit off. We couldn't hide it anymore. We told our parents and friends. We told Darryn. Two years later he started to use a cane. Toward the end of 1982 he got a pair of crutches, the kind with arm supports for more stability.

Then early in 1985, about ten years after he was diagnosed, Steven bought a motorized scooter to get around at work, in shopping malls, and other places where lots of walking was required. On one hand the scooter was a great relief to me. I no longer had to watch him struggle to walk a block. I no longer had to worry if he was going to fall and break his neck. The scooter gave us back some long-lost freedom. It made it easier to go places—as long as they were accessible. On the other hand the scooter was a reminder that the MS was here to stay, the unwanted, but permanent lodger in our home.

After numerous conversations with myself over the years, I had set a timetable for Steven's increasing disability that I thought I could live with. I accepted the possibility, even the probability, that he might end up in a wheelchair in his mid-fifties. When he needed one thirteen years ahead of my "schedule," extreme sadness mixed with a lot of hidden anger overtook me. As Steven became more and more disabled, I became a classic example of Freudian sublimation. I couldn't admit my pain or my anger so I channeled most of my energy into work-related activities instead. I concentrated on my career and was always so busy between work, being a mom, and being a homemaker, that I literally didn't have time to dwell on Steven's worsening physical condition.

But pushing myself didn't make the pain go away. It didn't resolve my grief. Instead it turned anger into anguish and then into major depression that required a long period of intensive therapy and medication before it ended, before I regained my mental and emotional equilibrium. For the first time since Steven came home from the hospital those many years before, I let myself cry and through my tears began to heal.

If you've never suffered from depression, or even spent time with someone who has, it is a very difficult disease to comprehend. The chemical imbalance that occurs in the brain during periods of major depression somehow causes feelings of dread, fear, and anxiety to take over. For me, depression appears as a dark menacing cloud directly over my head, even on a sunny day. The cloud is ominous and jagged, not fluffy and white. It bears down on me as if it were a heavy steel plate and makes it hard for me to stand up straight. The pain is unbearable, although it isn't a physical pain. All I want is for it to stop because life seems worthless if it won't go away. The pressure of the cloud on my head and back causes me to lose all my self-confidence. Making decisions, even very simple ones, such as whether to buy white bread or whole wheat, becomes unbearably difficult, and thus another source of pain and anguish. I lose my appetite during bouts of depression and can't sleep more than an hour or two at a time. The irony of it all is that all I seem to want to do during those times is get into bed and pull the covers over my head so I won't have to face the world, so I won't have to feel.

These bouts of depression, which began in 1986 and have come and gone three times since, are terrible for Steven. He feels so helpless in his wheelchair with his limited dexterity. But I tell him he is my lifeline, and if I didn't need to physically assist him every day, I might never make the effort to care for myself. I tell him that even though he can't really do anything for me physically, he gives me the emotional strength to fight the depression. At times like this I know how important it is to have someone who loves you close by. That is one of the key factors for me in getting well, but I also know I couldn't do it without medication and talk therapy, both of which help restore me to health. The medication works on the chemicals in my brain that are out of whack, and the talk therapy gives me the opportunity, the permission, to confront my demons and better understand them.

William Styron, the Pulitzer Prize-winning writer perhaps best known as the author of *Sophie's Choice* and *The*

Confessions of Nat Turner, suffered from depression. He wrote about his experience in the book *Darkness Visible: A Memoir of Madness*:

> *What I had begun to discover is that, mysteriously and in ways that are totally remote from normal experience, the gray drizzle of horror induced by depression takes on the quality of physical pain. But it is not an immediately identifiable pain, like that of a broken limb. It may be more accurate to say that despair, owing to some evil trick played upon the sick brain by the inhabiting psyche, comes to resemble the diabolical discomfort of being imprisoned in a fiercely overheated room. And because no breeze stirs this caldron, because there is no escape from this smothering confinement, it is entirely natural that the victim begins to think ceaselessly of oblivion.*

After Steven read the book he told me that although he had lived through periods of depression with me and saw it first hand, the book gave him an appreciation for what I was going through that he didn't have before, that he could not have imagined. Try as I might, I don't have a similar appreciation for the extreme and enervating fatigue that sometimes overtakes him without warning, or the anguish that causes him to scream in frustration when he tries to rise from his wheelchair with a big boost from me, but no matter how hard he tries he just can't get the lift he needs. I imagine the exhaustion. I see the struggle, but I know they are nothing compared to his reality.

There's a delicate balance between giving in, hanging on, and graciously accepting the inevitable. Steven and I had to learn to deal with these various reactions. We had to recognize that we tend to do things in very different ways. We learned that we needed to find a way to satisfy our competing grieving and coping styles. What ultimately got us back together, and has kept us together, is the recognition that, although he is the one with clinical MS, "we," the family Mintz, also have MS, at least in a psychosocial sense, and Steven's needs must be met, but so must mine.

Steven's a quiet fighter. He stretches his ability to the limit grabbing for each piece of independence he can preserve. Not wanting to let the MS get the upper hand he will struggle to maintain his current level of activity as long as possible. Even when he might have easily fallen down the stairs to the basement, when it was clearly beyond his ability to safely walk down, he would keep on even if it took him a half hour or forty-five minutes rather than admit defeat. I admire that greatly, but I ached inside each time I watched him struggle to do what most of us can do so easily. I didn't always admire this quality in him. In fact, I used to hate it because I thought he was just being stubborn, and sometimes even mean. I didn't appreciate that, like Don Quixote, fighting the invisible foe is what he needs to do to emotionally survive.

Steven and I have learned the hard way that understanding and accepting each other's inner needs, knowing each other's devils, is a great deal harder than understanding and accepting the realities of disability. But that when you do, you have a treasure to last you a lifetime.

Despite the fact that he now needs help with the standard activities of daily living (dressing, bathing, toileting, eating, mobility, and transferring from bed to wheelchair, etc.), our lives are good for the time being. We share the things we always have: going to the movies and the theatre; reading mysteries; doing crossword puzzles; listening to jazz; eating good food; and our latest joint activity, Sudoku, the Japanese logic puzzle that seems to have popped up out of nowhere and become an obsession of ours and so many others over night. We miss dancing and "standing-up hugs," the latter probably more than anything, but we are grateful that Steven is still working, and full time at that. Twice a week a neighbor drives Steven to work at the Department of Energy in Washington, DC, in our specially modified minivan with its built-in ramp and electric doors. We've been very fortunate to have neighbors who work near Steven and are willing to help out. The other three days he telecommutes by computer from our home. (Thank heaven for modern technology.) When the first edition of this book was published in 2002, Steven was still driving himself, but the MS continued its relentless attack on his body and deciding to stop driving was a really big decision, as I am sure you can imagine. On the upbeat side of life, Darryn is all grown up. She's married and has made us grandparents, which is as great an experience as everyone always says it is. And they live only ten minutes away, which makes it even better.

I don't know what sort of a person I would have turned into without the tragedies that befell Steven and me, but I do know that I have done things and have an approach to life now that I never could have imagined if our lives had been easier. I am glad for my added character, my achievements, my compassion, but I would trade all of it in a heartbeat if it meant that I could wake up one morning to find Steven well.

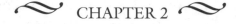

CHAPTER 2

The Common Bonds
of Caregiving

On a bright and sunny weekend in September of 1991 after school had reopened and the vacationers had left the beach, but while the weather was still delightfully warm, I went away for the weekend with my long-time friend Cindy Fowler. We went for a respite from the pressure of our lives.

Cindy was caring for her seventy-eight-year-old mother, Madeleine, who was suffering from Parkinson's disease. She'd moved from Kansas City and lived somewhat independently in the small apartment above the Fowler's garage, but soon moved into the spare bedroom in the Fowler's house. Madeleine had been living with Cindy, her husband Rich, their thirteen-year-old son, Chris, and their foster son Huong for three years when Cindy and I went off for our weekend fling.

Steven had significant mobility problems by then. He'd been using a scooter for a number of years to get around out of doors, but moving around in the house was starting to become difficult as well. He could still get in and out of bed, dress himself, and take care of his other personal needs, albeit slowly and by holding on to walls and counter tops in the process, but for all intents and purposes you could say he was able to function independently inside the house. The fact that his disability was, and is to this day, only physical meant I knew he could make wise decisions should something out of the ordinary occur. Under those circumstances I could go away for the weekend without worrying a great deal and without needing to make elaborate arrangements for his care.

And so we went, leaving after work on a Friday evening and looking forward to a pleasant three-and-a-half-hour drive to Dewey Beach, Delaware, and the beach house of a friend who had graciously lent it to me for the weekend. But about an hour into the drive we hit stop-and-go traffic that soon turned into a complete standstill because of what we later learned was a very serious accident up ahead, an accident so serious that it required Medivac helicopters to transport injured people to a trauma center in Baltimore.

As night came on and we were sitting in the dark, closed environment of the car we began to talk to each other in a way we never had before. Cindy was a very private person at that time in her life. I didn't often know much about her inner thoughts, her hidden worries, but that night in the intimacy of the close quarters of the car she opened up and began talking about her concerns regarding Madeleine, about the difficulty of getting helpful information, about the emotional and growing physical impact caring for her mom was having on her. She knew my story fairly well. She had seen Steven deteriorating over the years, and she and her husband Rich were the first friends Steven told that he had MS. She knew the emotional pressures that the MS had caused in our lives, about our separations, and about my early bouts with depression. But despite this we had never talked about our fears, asked each other practical questions about providing care, or recognized that there were similarities in our situations. That night we did.

It was as if the proverbial light bulb went on, and it stayed on that entire weekend. As we sat on the beach and soaked up the sun, as we sat on the screened porch of the house after dinner and sipped a cup of coffee, and as we drove home in the light of day on Sunday afternoon we talked, asked each other questions, discussed our concerns about the future, and realized that although Cindy was caring for her mom, and I was assisting my husband, that although Madeleine was elderly and had Parkinson's disease, and Steven was still in his forties and had MS, we were feeling the same anguish, the same emotional distress, and were concerned about similar issues. And we wondered why it seemed that no one recognized these similarities. We wondered why no one seemed to be focused on the fact that helping a loved one with a deteriorating illness had a very real impact on not only the person with the illness, but also on those of us who were primarily responsible for helping them.

We somehow knew the term *family caregiver*, although neither of us could say when we had first heard it, but know it we did, and now recognized that despite the differences between our circumstances it applied to us equally. We were family caregivers, not solely of course, but caregiving was a very real part of who we were, and we wanted people to take notice. We were family caregivers, and we wanted someone to reach out to us, to tell us where to find helpful information and advice, emotional support, and real hands-on assistance when we needed it. We weren't looking for, nor did we want, a pat on the back because we were caring for a family member we dearly loved, but we did want recognition of the difficulties involved. We wanted these things but as far as we knew they didn't exist, or if they did, they weren't readily available.

We had been good friends before but now we recognized this common bond. We now instinctively knew that we were not alone, that there must be thousands more people like us, thousands more family caregivers, needing what we needed, sharing common concerns, feeling the same emotions, needing much of the same kind of help and information. That spark of recognition is what ignited our desire to do something, but do what we did not know.

Cindy is a graphic designer and the vice president of her own award-winning design firm, Graves Fowler Associates. At the time, I was the principal in charge of marketing for a leading interior architectural firm in Washington, DC. Cindy knew how to design a newsletter. I was itching to do some writing separate and apart from what I did as part of my job. At some point during the ride home from the beach, the idea to try and create a newsletter for family caregivers was hatched, a newsletter that spoke to the common needs and concerns of family caregivers, regardless of whether they were caring for a spouse, a parent, a child, or a sibling, and regardless of what disease or disability their loved one had.

We didn't have a grand plan, just pent-up emotion, an idea, and a desire to make a difference. And thus we began. I wrote the articles. Cindy did the design, and through her professional connections we were able to have the first news-letter, all four pages of it, printed for free. We called the news-letter *TAKE CARE! Self Care for the Family Caregiver*, and thus began our journey.

We made contact with the social work department of local hospitals, met with a number of voluntary health agen-cies (that's the official name for groups such as the Alzheimer's Association, the National Multiple Sclerosis Society, and the American Cancer Society). We showed them the newsletter and asked them to share it with others. We requested indi-viduals to give us $5.00 if they wanted to receive future issues by mail.

A respite weekend at the beach. Two friends sharing the intimacy of time away together. Thoughts and feelings are expressed, an idea is born, and a toe is put into the water of the lake of good intentions to test the temperature of our commitment and capabilities. The temperature must have been right on because two years later, in the spring of 1993, *TAKE CARE!* became the official publication of the newly formed National Family Caregivers Association (NFCA).

Much has happened since those tentative days. NFCA has grown and changed. I am proud to say that today it is recognized as the leading organization for family caregivers, and the only one speaking with the authentic voice of experi-ence. As you would expect, NFCA reaches out to family caregivers across the life span and the boundaries of differing diagnoses and relationships to address the common needs and concerns of all family caregivers. The organization's mission is:

> *to empower family caregivers to act on behalf of themselves and their loved ones and remove barriers to health and wellbeing.*

And our vision is of:

> *an America in which family caregivers lead full and productive lives, free from depression, pain, isolation, and financial distress.*

We strive to accomplish our mission and realize our vision by providing education, support, and a public voice for America's family caregivers so that all caregiving families can have a better quality of life. If you would like to find out more about NFCA and become part of our caregiving community, visit our Web site www.thefamilycaregiver.org or call 1-800-896-3650.

The Weaver's Thread

What are those common bonds of caregiving that Cindy and I discovered during that wonderful respite weekend at the beach? What is the single thread that ties together those of us who care for spouses, children, parents, siblings, partners, or friends who are chronically ill, frail, or disabled?

The common thread certainly isn't the tasks of caregiving. They vary so much, from helping a developmentally delayed child learn new skills, to taking an aging parent to frequent doctor's appointments, to turning a bed-ridden spouse every few hours day and night. The tasks of caregiving can differ tremendously from situation to situation.

It surely isn't the number of years involved. Caregiving can last a few short months, as when you are caring for a terminal cancer patient. It can last three to five years when caring for an aged parent who has a weak heart. At times, caregiving can be a lifetime commitment for a family, especially when a severely disabled child is involved.

Location varies from situation to situation. Although the vast majority of caregiving goes on in the home and many caregivers and recipients live under the same roof, talk to anyone whose parent is in a nursing home, or whose child lives in a group home, and you'll quickly learn that caregiving doesn't end when someone else is responsible for day-to-day care, or when caregiving takes place across long distances. Different situations have different demands and require different capabilities and commitments from us.

If it isn't the responsibilities or tasks, and it is not the length of time or the location, what is the essential bond of family caregiving? What does caring for a spouse with heart disease have to do with caring for parents who are losing their ability to live independently, or a child with spinabifida?

If you read caregivers' letters, if you listen to their stories as I have, it is very clear that the common bond between all caregivers is its emotional impact. Listen to these statements. Can you tell whether they were written by a spouse, or a parent, a partner, a loving friend, a sibling, an adult child or grandchild, or someone in another caregiving relationship? Can you tell which disease or disability their loved one has?

> *I feel overwhelmed most of the time and accomplish very little except meeting our immediate needs.*

> *I have nurses during the day to care for _____ so I can work and I have nurses at night so I can sleep. . . . I have NO time to care for myself.*

> *I think watching someone you love so much deteriorate is really more stress than anything in the world.*

All three of these quotes express some of the common experiences of family caregivers: feeling overwhelmed, loss of all personal time, and sadness and stress. The wife of a stroke victim wrote the first one. The mother of a severely disabled child wrote the second, and a young woman who cares for her grandmother wrote the last one.

There are certainly differences in each caregiving circumstance. A caregiver helping an elderly aunt who has diabetes will be dealing with different issues than a caregiver whose spouse has Lou Gehrig's Disease (ALS). These are the differences of our individual day-to-day realities and they are very real indeed. The things that separate us are the names of our loved one's diagnosis and the specific parts of the body or mind that the condition attacks.

Steven has a physical disability, but his mind is clear. The struggles of our day-to-day existence involve mobility issues, toileting, and the tasks that healthy hands usually perform. Getting in and out of bed, buttoning shirts, the height of toilets, catheterization, and making sure the batteries that power his wheelchair are fully charged, these are our concerns. But my friend Judy had to deal with a very different set of daily circumstances when she cared for her husband who had Alzheimer's disease. Helping him remember the day of the week and what was said five minutes ago, making sure the doors had special locks so he couldn't wander away and get lost, trying to balance caring for him and being available for her three children at the same time were the issues she struggled with. These are the day-to-day realities of caring for someone with a specific diagnosis.

These are very real differences, as is the fact that a wife obviously has a very different relationship with her spouse than a daughter has with her father. Your spouse is your peer, your partner, your lover. Your father helped give you life and taught you how to live it. He taught you how to ride a bike and read you a book at night. These are the specific circumstances of relationship that affect our caregiving lives. But beneath these layers of variations, at the core of caregiving, lie the common bond of feelings that so many family caregivers share.

I may not know what it is like to have two disabled children as my friend Nan does, but nevertheless we share similar feelings. We both know the isolation that so many caregivers describe. We can relate to the frustration that comes with caregiving, and we both know the changes, large and small, that transform our relationships in disturbing ways. We both know the sadness that comes from watching someone we love struggle to do what is a simple task for most of us. We are both very aware of the vast distance between the realities of our world and what the able-bodied, healthy world thinks of as normal, but we also both know the love we feel that sees past the problems we face, the inner strength we never could have imagined we had, and a view of life that is both filled with compassion and a focus on the beauty and importance of human dignity. These are the common bonds of caregiving.

Isolation

The isolation that comes from having to put so much focus on what the professionals call "activities of daily living" is compounded when friends and family turn away. So many caregivers are literally isolated from others.

> *A lot of people don't want to be around someone who is sick. Some friends may never call or stop by again.*
> —Josh Sparber, Anaheim, CA

I've often wondered what it is about caregiving situations that frighten our friends away, and I've decided it is that our lives are a mirror in which they see what could possibly happen to them and their loved ones, and because the reflection is scary they turn away. They don't know how to react in our presence, what to talk about, how to be with us. We can't do the things we used to do. We are less mobile, less socially nimble. Perhaps a brain injury means our spouse is no longer a charming conversationalist, or our sister has spasms and cannot talk clearly. We can't do things on the spur of the moment anymore now that Mom is living with us and can't be left alone.

No one wants to think about adversity. No one wants to see it staring him or her in the face. And yet that is what

people need to do if they are going to be our friends. They
will have to put their fears aside and learn how to maneuver a
wheelchair and possibly learn how to communicate with us in
a new way. That's why they are friends, and we will cherish
them all the more for sticking by us because we know that so
many others have a hard time dealing with our changed situation and will drift away.

Diffusing Awkwardness

One way to try to prevent friends from drifting away is to
learn how to make people comfortable with your new situation. If your loved one's problems are strictly physical, perhaps he would like to be the one to explain to others exactly
what is going on in his body, what limitations his condition
causes and why. Fear of the unknown, discomfort with not
knowing the proper way to act or what to say to someone
who is different is one of the reasons that others feel awkward
around us.

I recall one time when Steven and I went to see our niece
Alisa, an amateur actress, perform in a play in Baltimore. Steven
was using a scooter at the time, and we drove a small station
wagon that allowed us to easily store the scooter in the back.
After the show Alisa, her husband George, and some of their
friends, who had also come to see the show that night, walked
us to our car. They helped dismantle the scooter and put it in
the back of the wagon and then stood around not knowing
what else to do or say. Often in those days Steven's legs would
go into spasm when he tried to get into the car. He'd manage
to get his duff down onto the passenger seat but his legs would
stiffen and shoot out in front of him, so that he was sitting
facing the door instead of the hood of the car with his legs
stiff and straight as wooden boards.

As I tried to break the spasm so he could bend his knees
and pivot to the left and be in position for me to lift his legs
up and into the car, he calmly explained to the young people
standing around exactly what happened and why his legs went
into spasm. He told them about MS and how it stripped the

nerves of their protective coating and how the scar tissue that replaced it made it very difficult, and sometimes impossible, for instructions from his brain to reach the muscles in his legs. They all listened attentively as he talked to them, and as his legs slowly lost their stiffness and became more flexible I picked them up one at a time and put them on the floor of the car as he pivoted his body so he was at last fully settled in the passenger seat, all the time keeping up the explanation. There was no awkwardness and no silent staring, which so often happens when people see someone who is disabled. The kids asked questions and you could see that they lost their initial uneasiness because of Steven's openness. I was so proud of him and how he diffused an embarrassing situation and transformed it into both an educational and comfortable one for everyone. I knew from that point onward George and Alisa would never feel awkward around us no matter how disabled Steven became, and I was right.

It Is Hard, But—

It is important to try to maintain social contacts when you are a family caregiver because it is so easy for caregiving to be all consuming. There is a book about Alzheimer's caregiving called *The 36 Hour Day*. That title is a good example of just how full your life can become when you add caregiving to an already busy schedule. Layer on top of that the physical and emotional energy-drain that difficult caregiving days can bring and it is clear why we often don't have the energy to go out and party. Resting at home may well seem far more restorative than making the effort to dress and dine out with friends, and yet doing normal fun things like that is what keeps us connected, both with friends and the world beyond caregiving.

The loneliness of caregiving is ironic. We need time and energy to socialize and that's exactly what is in shortest supply when you are a family caregiver. One way to combat that is to have a friend give you a call at a scheduled time every few days or once a week. That way you are in touch with someone who cares, and since you know when the call is going to come in you can arrange other activities around it.

But as comforting as phone calls can be, caregivers do also need to get out of the house. If you are a working caregiver your job may not only help pay bills, but also fulfill part of your need to socialize with others. If you can find a neighbor to go power walking you can combine exercise and a chat, two things that are good for you, for the price of one. Perhaps just knowing that isolation is a likely and debilitating consequence of caregiving can help you be alert enough to take steps to prevent it from getting a hold on your heart and on your life. No one ever said that life is fair, but hopefully we don't have to add the pain of isolation to our woes if we can take steps to avoid it.

Feelings of Frustration

I feel agitation, frustration, and guilt that I can't always be the victorious overcoming person I long to be.
—Evelyn M. Nichols, Cedaredge, OH

I get so frustrated when he awakens me several times a night because his hallucinations are real to him.
—Anna Shank, Hanover, PA

Another common bond of caregiving is the frustration we all experience because it is so hard to get things done, because non-caregivers just don't understand, because healthy people park in handicapped parking spots, and because our healthcare system isn't designed to respond to the needs of people with chronic conditions. Frustrations abound at every turn.

My friend, Evie, who was a highly resourceful caregiver for her husband before he passed away, says she reached her frustration limit when equipment broke or didn't function the way it was supposed to. Evie tells the story of the company sales rep who told her over the phone that the lifts his company manufactured to help transfer a non-mobile person from bed to wheelchair never break, while she stood there in her bedroom with a broken bolt in her hand and the lift in pieces on the floor. "My first reaction was to scream at the guy," she said, "but then I realized I would get more help if I didn't rant and rave, but rather told him in no uncertain terms how I needed him to fix my problem."

It isn't possible to get rid of all the frustrations in our lives, whether we are a caregiver or not, but a way I have found to lessen my frustration is to decide what is really worth getting upset about and what isn't. A former colleague of mine named Jim had a great way of making you think about what was really important and what was not. He'd ask, "Is it worth falling on your sword for?" What a powerful way to say pick your priorities. If we are going to let every inconvenience and snub get under our skin, we'll constantly be frustrated. Better to decide where to put our psychic energy and what to let go of.

One of the things that frustrates me is the inconsiderateness of healthcare professionals especially because they should know better. Time and again when Steven goes to a doctor we are left to figure out on our own how to get him up on the examining table. They see Steven in his wheelchair and know that he can't maneuver on his own, but nevertheless do nothing to help. They just walk out of the room. I then have to go and find some people to assist us, and there aren't always appropriate people around. It would be nice if they figured out how to accommodate people who are wheelchair bound. Fortunately our family doctor, Steve Schwartz, has, which is one of the reasons we chose him. Forward thinking in many ways, his medical records are electronic, he welcomes e-mail, and his practice recently purchased an adjustable exam table to better serve Steven and other disabled or elderly patients. The cost difference was less than $1,000 and the IRS provides a 50 percent disability tax credit to make it even more affordable. You have to wonder why other physician offices aren't taking advantage of this win/win opportunity. I have to believe they just don't know about it.

Another of my hot buttons is the same as Evie's—equipment problems. Because we rely so completely on Steven's power wheelchair in order to have a life, we are both thrown into a tizzy when it isn't working right. One way we've found to counteract this particular frustration is to find a very reliable home medical equipment company. The company we use actually sends a technician out to the house to fix the problem right there—a doctor for wheelchairs who makes house calls. It doesn't stop the fact that something can go wrong, but it does give us confidence that the problem will be fixed, and with as little hassle as possible.

I could make a whole list of the things that frustrate me, including at times Steven, but I purposely try to keep my list short. After all you can't go down on your sword every time someone is inconsiderate or the doctor didn't provide the pharmacy with your mom's prescription reauthorization on the day she said she would, thereby necessitating an extra trip. No, we can't remove frustration from our lives (if we could we'd be living in Eden) but we can try to lessen its hold on us. One way is to plan ahead; another is to think about the most serious of our problems and try to find solutions that will at least make them shrink and ideally go away altogether.

Frustration is an exhausting emotion. It enervates us, takes away our equilibrium. The only way it can have a positive effect on our lives is if it prods us to get rid of its cause. Since there is no way we can always do that, remember to pick your battles and decide what issues are worth expending energy on. That might help you feel less like a wounded warrior, more of the time.

Changing Family Dynamics

My role as a wife has changed to Mommy of a once humorous, bright, and articulate husband.
                              —Susan Kiser Scarff, Phoenix, AZ

What's the hardest thing about being a family caregiver? Changing roles from being the child to being the one in control.

—Anna Shank, Hanover, PA

The upheaval of changing family dynamics that occurs because life has been turned upside down is something that all family caregivers can relate to. The changing relationships often catch us off guard. We spend so much time and energy dealing with the tasks of caregiving, getting over emotional shock, or grieving our losses that we often don't see how our caregiving responsibilities are taking time away from the other people we love. The relationship does usually change between caregiver and care receiver, but it can also change between us and our friends and siblings and a host of others as well. The dynamics that accompany the decline in someone's health or a sudden change in circumstances are complex and disturbing. It's no wonder that we don't recognize them until they've caused a rift and are getting in the way, not only of our ability to be effective caregivers, but also of our very happiness.

Not all the changing family dynamics in caregiving families are negative; some surveys have found that caregivers and care recipients build closer bonds. In some families there is an initial ripping apart followed by a new closeness. Regardless of whether the effects are negative or positive, or a combination of both, the fact that caregiving affects family relationships cannot be denied.

My daughter moved home [to help with caregiving for her dad]. This is a big help because she is very aware of how I feel and the need for me to talk. She has been a wonderful source of support.

—Frances Rouse, Streetsboro, OH

My mom and I started to grow closer some years ago after she became a caregiver for my dad. He had a stroke that left him incontinent, slightly demented, and with exaggerated embarrassing tendencies, such as a penchant for taking things from the local Office Depot. Mom and I began to speak virtually every day as compared to our traditional pattern of once a week. She'd ask my advice. She would pour out her heart, tell me about her fear and her embarrassment over my dad's actions. I would try to comfort her and make what I hoped were helpful suggestions. I arranged homecare for Steven so I could go to Florida and physically be with her and my dad more often. We conversed on a level we never had before, very much peer to peer, each having a better understanding of the other's personality and the other's pain than we ever could have if we both weren't caregivers.

A few years ago when I went through a particularly difficult bout of depression, she sent me a greeting card every day, sometimes twice a day, to remind me I was loved, to tell me I was special, to let me know that there would be brighter days ahead. I kept them all on the mantle, even when they were stacked three deep until she came for a visit. I wanted her to know how much I appreciated them, how much they helped. My dad is now gone and Mom has more freedom to come and visit. I enjoy her company when she is here. We are still very definitely mother and daughter, but in some ways we are sisters too, and I kind of like that.

Some people talk about role reversal when referring to a situation in which an adult child is caring for her parent, but I think that's wrong. We aren't reversing our roles. We aren't really becoming our parents' parent. We are helping them as they age in ways they used to help us, but if they have all of their faculties we must remember they have the right to make their own decisions, whether we agree with them or not. We can guide and advise them. They can ask more of us than they ever did in the past, and we can see them in a weakened condition that is antithetical to the image we had of them when we were kids, but we can never change the fact that they are our parents and we are their children.

The changing nature of relationships in caregiving situations is a touchy one. Can you still view your husband as a lover if you have to wipe his bottom every day? Can you still love your sister if she refuses to help care for your mother, especially if you are making many sacrifices to do so yourself? Will your marriage survive the pain of having produced a child with mental retardation? Will the other kids accept and love their new sister, even though she is different? These are very difficult questions. They force us to confront the very fabric of who we are as human beings. They test our compassion and our commitment and our feelings for another. Burying them under a rug will not make them go away. We do need to examine them, perhaps go into therapy individually or as a family, to help us deal with them. Unfortunately they won't just go away on their own.

The On-going Sadness and Grief of Caregivers

Perhaps the two most difficult aspects of caregiving to deal with are the on-going sadness and grief that haunt caregivers' lives and the different realities of caregiving families and non-caregiving families.

One of the most difficult emotions involved with caregiving is the intense sadness we feel because we love someone whose life is challenging, who hasn't been given the same chance as others, whose vigor has been taken away, or whose mental functioning has deteriorated. One of the common bonds of caregiving is the sadness that comes from wanting the miracle of wellness.

> *My daughter was born with such limiting disabilities that I have had to give up every dream I ever had for her.*
> —Esther McGee, Monroe, LA

The sadness of family caregivers cuts to the core of who we are as people because it touches on true grief and it ebbs and flows through our lives, sometimes right at the surface and other times buried far below. Learning to manage our

sadness and grieving our losses is something that all caregivers
need to learn how to do.

In one of her syndicated columns, author Ellen Goodman
talked about an unwritten schedule of grief, the fact that we
Americans expect things to happen quickly, that we have no
patience for problems that linger, for wounds that do not
heal. She said:

> *The American way of dealing with it [grief], however,
> has turned grieving into a set process with rules, stages,
> and of course deadlines. We have, in essence, tried to
> make a science of grief, to tuck messy emotions under
> neat clinical labels—like "survivor guilt" or "detach-
> ment."* . . .*We expect, maybe insist upon, an end to
> grief. Trauma, pain, detachment, acceptance in a year.
> Time's up. But in real lives, grief is a train that doesn't
> run on anyone else's schedule.*

What do we do with this caregiver grief that never fully
goes away, that doesn't have a terminus, and that may, from
time to time, spring afresh with new tears and new fears? We
need to acknowledge it for one thing. There's no reason to
deny its existence. Call it by its name. Our feelings are our
feelings. They are an essential part of us. Burying them only
makes them change from seeds, which our tears can nourish
and nurture so we can see them for what they are, into a
festering mold that stays tucked away inside and eats at our
inner core.

Denying our grief denies our humanity. If we didn't care,
we wouldn't feel so bad. So I suggest, take out the tissues,
share your sorrow with a friend and with your loved one, if
you can. Be good to yourself. Find emotional nourishment;
get lots of hugs. Grieving is hard work. It takes time and
energy. Learn from the experience so that hopefully you can
grow from it, so that the grief doesn't debilitate you.

It's been more than thirty years since Steven was first diagnosed with MS. I have dreamed new dreams. I have laughed.

We have experienced the goodness of life. But sometimes the old wound aches in a certain way and I know, as I believe all family caregivers know, that I am in for a spell.

When your wound hurts, whether it is still fresh or seemingly healed beneath scar tissue as mine is, remember Ellen Goodman's words: "Hearts heal faster from surgery than from loss" and know that it is okay to cry, for yourself as well as for your loved one.

Sadness and the need to grieve are two of the bonds that tie all family caregivers together. To help express these feelings and come to terms with them, some family caregivers write poetry. Sometimes they send their poetry to NFCA, and I am given the privilege of seeing inside another human being's heart.

Rita Cassidy Wiggins a caregiver for her husband with Alzheimer's disease wrote a poem titled "Discovery." In it she expressed the gradual grief of caregiving, the inner pain and the sadness that accompanied the progression of his disease.

> *How subtly it intrudes,*
> *this gradual grief*
> *seldom visible to others,*
> *careful not to summon tears.*
> *Sometimes it seems to slip away,*
> *leaving just a shadow,*
> *barely there.*
> *Until one ordinary day,*
> *you look up and sadness is everywhere.*

Jean Saucer, a caregiver for her son with mental illness, wrote about the pain of lost dreams and the randomness with which illness strikes.

> *I had dreams too*
> *confiscated by storms*
> *and human love.*
> *Reduced to silence*

by no one's greed,
but by the winds of chance.
I dance in the spring rain
a lightning rod for thunder's pain.

Not happy poems these, but poems that reflect true feelings that family caregivers experience, feelings aroused by circumstances that are outside most people's realities.

A Different Reality

Peter Dickinson is one of my favorite authors. He writes mysteries, but they are always more than mysteries. They are beautifully crafted stories that shed light on the human experience, stories that make you stop and reread a sentence two or three more times before you are willing to leave it there on the page and move on.

In his book, *Some Deaths Before Dying*, there is a sentence I've never been able to forget, perhaps because it was said by the lead character, a woman who was dying from a degenerative muscle disease and at the time of the story was bedridden, able to just move her eyelids and speak only haltingly. She had been a vibrant woman who in her healthier years had to some extent been a caregiver for her husband who had been a prisoner of war during World War II and came home bearing psychological scars. In referring to what had happened to her husband, and therefore to herself she thought, "She too had been betrayed by happenings beyond her sphere, and now she was expected to live and behave like a normal citizen, despite that." The sentence took my breath away. Indeed, isn't that what happened to all of us who answer to the title of family caregiver. Isn't that what happened to the spouses, parents, partners, friends, children, siblings for whom we care? We've "been betrayed by happenings" we couldn't control and presented with the daunting challenge of trying to re-create normalcy.

It isn't an easy thing to do, re-create normalcy when you've been hit by what feels like the equivalent of an atomic blast, and yet that is what is expected of us, and indeed what we always strive to do. But I have come to realize that for my family and other caregiving families, normalcy is very different than it is for families that don't have to deal with disability, with the almost perverse attention to the basic acts of life that come with it and the myriad arrangements we must make to do ordinary things.

I recall once seeing a young man walking down the street. He was a wearing the typical costume of his generation, jeans and a T-shirt. Blazoned across the front of his chest in bold black letters was the statement "Normal Is Boring." I read it as he passed by me and I thought to myself, "He doesn't have a clue. He doesn't realize that normal isn't boring at all. It is the most wonderful thing in the world." Normal is what those of us who are family caregivers want more than anything else. We want to be like other families that take walking and talking and eating and toileting and swallowing and thinking for granted. We want our loved ones to be well. No, normal isn't boring at all, except perhaps to those who have never experienced the outside-the-norm situations of caregiving.

Steven and I have a definition of normalcy that fits our current circumstances, a definition that inevitably changes over time, as his MS continues to take its toll and impact our collective lives. These days our definition of normal includes the fact that Steven still has some strength in his legs and arms and therefore can be an active participant in helping me help him with transfers, showering, dressing, toileting, and eating. When the time comes when he can no longer do that, we will need to find other ways to deal with these basic life activities. Most likely we will need to get a lift of some sort. Regardless of what decisions we make down the road, the new situation we will be living with will, by definition, become our norm, at least after the transition period from the old way of doing things to the new way is completed. What normal means for Steven and I is most likely quite different from your definition, especially if your caregiving situation is not the same as ours. How we each define normalcy isn't important, but what is important is finding a way to comfortably live with the norms that are now part of our lives, and recognize that in the world of a caregiver what's normal today may no longer be what you consider normal a year from now.

I haven't decided whether it is easier to redefine normalcy when the changes come gradually or when they come because of a more dramatic occurrence. Certainly gradual change is easier to assimilate into our lives, but it lacks the clarity of catastrophe, and doesn't always give us the opportunity to recognize the change for what it is because it sort of oozes its way slowly into our lives. But regardless of whether the changes come swiftly or slowly, they play havoc with our emotions, and we are forced to deal with what I have come to think of as the bridge between anger and acceptance.

Anger and Acceptance

Anger is an emotion we have been taught to try to hide, but these days I think of it as a very healthy emotion, one that reminds us that we are very much alive and that we burn with the fire of desire for the good things of life. Expressing our anger at the difficulties we face, the indignities we must endure, at the complex arrangements we have to make to do what should be simple tasks done by rote, is healthy. To rail at the gods is okay—for a time. But anger that is continuous, that can't be soothed, that lies buried beneath a calm exterior and festers like a dirty wound isn't healthy. Anger must eventually give way, move beyond itself to acceptance of our situation, not placid acceptance that saps our energy, but a dynamic acceptance that translates into actions that help us make the most of our transformed lives.

How do we do that? I don't know that there is one set way. We must each find our own answers to that question. I can tell you about my own experience and hopefully there will be something in it that you can grab onto to help you move beyond any anger you may be harboring. For me it is about conscious decision making, about making choices. Chapter four, "Building Confidence and Capabilities:

Making Choices, Taking Charge" explores this concept in some detail, but let me say here that for me crossing the bridge from anger to acceptance is about consciously saying, and believing, that this is where I want to be. It is about choosing to take on the responsibility of caregiving. To me, that is very different than believing that I am forced to be a caregiver. I believe that despite the difficulties we confront, life awaits us. For sure it challenges us, more than it does the families of the able bodied and mentally fit. We all wish it would challenge us less, but it is the palette of colors we have been given, and the artistry of our lives is defined by the picture we create with our "other than normal" assortment of crayons. I am not saying it is easy. It is to be sure a crooked path, a wobbly bridge, and I have no idea what lies around the next bend, but I am no longer feeling that I was forced to be on this path, and that's the difference. Like the Robert Frost poem in which two paths converge in a wood, I am choosing to walk on the one less traveled. I am choosing to be a family caregiver.

My life has been "betrayed by happenings beyond my sphere" and for many years I could not accept that. But I slowly crossed the bridge and consciously chose to accept my new reality, and now with open eyes I act very purposefully and strive to "live and behave like a normal citizen." And I invite you to do the same, to recognize the emotions that caregiving has evoked in you, to embrace the inner strength that comes from dealing successfully with difficult situations, and to try to move beyond the frustration, the sadness, the isolation, and the other difficult emotions that so often come with being a family caregiver. Try to look inside yourself to see if you are harboring anger, as I was. If you can recognize it, you might just be able to use that energy in a more positive way to be proactive and take charge of your life.

A Life of Hope and Meaning

Although we hear the most about the dark side of caregiving it has untold rewards as well that are best expressed in caregivers' own words.

What makes caregiving rewarding for me is the smile on his face when I walk into his room. . . . As exhausting as it is for me to be his nurse, his social worker, his advocate, and his mom, all it takes to re-energize me is a few minutes at his side. Tyler's gentle caring of ME helps make it all worthwhile. He lays his hand upon my head and strokes my hair. It is calming and I think he likes being able to be the giver of care instead of the receiver.
—C. Robbins-Brady, Grand Junction, Colorado

As my caregiving responsibilities increased, I came to understand and accept many lessons as blessings in disguise. . . . Most of all I came to realize that caring for Sam is life itself—that nothing I can read or study, nothing I can talk about—nothing is as important or real as simply being present with him right here, right now.
—Phyllis Major, Palm Desert, California

Caregiving is a mixed bag when it comes to our emotions. So many of the emotions associated with caregiving are dark, as you have seen, but the wonderful thing about human beings is that most of us find a hidden well of capability, strength, and resolve we never knew we had, and more often than not, we have the resiliency that teaches us how to smile through our tears.

In the end, no matter how tired, scared, or worried I feel at times, I would not trade these past few years with my mother for anything. She has taught me the incredible gift of patience, acceptance, faith, and love.
—Liz McLeod, Kensington, Maryland

Things to Think About
What feelings and emotions do you associate with your caregiving experience—frustration, sadness, grief, love,

kindness, compassion, anger, pride, or guilt? Have you talked to other people about them, your loved one, a therapist, another family member or friend, another family caregiver perhaps? Talking about your feelings with others can really help you understand them better.

Have you thought about putting your thoughts down on paper, either in a poem or in a journal? Writing poetry and journaling are both good ways to get in touch with the emotions that caregiving arouses. They help us get underneath the crust we sometimes form as a protective coating against these emotions. Personal poems and journals don't have to be shared with anyone else. They can be your own private record of your inner self. They aren't about winning the Pulitzer Prize. They are about coming to terms with the life that the winds of chance have blown your way.

Recognize that you are not alone. There are millions of other family caregivers in America, more than fifty million in fact, that have the same thoughts and feelings that we do. There is no reason to be ashamed or embarrassed about any of your feelings. Remember that the emotions you feel are the common threads that tie you to others who care for a loved one who is chronically ill, disabled, or aged.

CHAPTER 3

"It Doesn't Have to Be This Hard"

There are other common bonds between family caregivers in addition to the emotions we all feel, and I alluded to them in the introduction. They are the difficulties we all face because our healthcare, social support systems, and employment and financial policies are not family-caregiver friendly. How would our lives, and our loved ones lives, be different if there was more alignment between the needs of caregiving families and the structure of our society? What if family caregiving was fully acknowledged and accepted as a societal issue that was everyone's problem and not just something for the families involved to handle? "Societal issue?" You might be asking, "What are you talking about? Caregiving is something that happens within a family." And you'd be right. Caregiving is something that happens within a family, but it also exists outside of it and beyond it.

In this day and age, caregiving is very much a social issue, and thankfully it is recognized as such a great deal more than it was when this book was first published in 2002. Today it is of concern to policy makers and politicians at the local, state, and federal level; employers; insurers; and healthcare providers. It is a topic of discussion in faith communities and the subject of evermore scientific and survey research. A study by Evercare and the National Alliance for Caregiving published in 2006, on the health risks of caring for a loved one, found that

> *the worry and stress of caregiving leads millions of caregivers to neglect their own physical and mental health, resulting in depression, extreme fatigue, poor eating and exercise habit and greater use of medications. More than half (fifty three percent) surveyed said this downward health spiral also negatively affects their ability to provide care.*

Today caregiving is much more than a personal family issue. It is the issue of our age because it will sooner or later affect every family in America, and we are not prepared either as individuals or as a society to deal with it.

Giving Care Isn't New—Caregiving Is

Families have always taken care of their ill or disabled loved ones. Neighbors helped neighbors if they didn't have family around, and even communities helped care for the ill among them, but the nature of giving care has changed radically. In the past

- Families didn't provide care for as many years as we do.
- Families didn't care for loved ones who are as ill, aged, or disabled as we do.
- Families didn't live in a highly mobile society as we do.
- Families didn't care for loved ones when so many women were employed and waited until their thirties or early forties to have children.
- Families didn't provide care at a time when healthcare costs and the question of who should pay for them were such an issue of concern.
- Families didn't provide care at a time when medical science had unlocked the secrets of the human genome

and knew how to save and extend lives in ways that were previously unimaginable.
- Families didn't care for loved ones at a time when the average age of the population was on the rise and baby boomers had already started turning sixty.

It is for all these reasons that caregiving is very different today than it ever was before. It is because of all these changes that have occurred in a relatively short period of time that the word *caregiver* even exists. The first recorded use of it was in 1975, according to *Merriam-Webster's Collegiate Dictionary*. The term *family caregiver* still hasn't made it into the tenth edition of that dictionary, and it was published in 2004.

I don't know about you, but I find it rather disconcerting that family caregivers don't even exist as far as the arbiters of American English are concerned, despite the fact that over 50 million people a year provide some level of care to an ill, aged, or disabled family member. References to family doctors go back as far as 1846 and the relatively new term *family practice*, sometimes referred to as *family medicine*, showed up in 1969.

> *It makes me very sad that nobody really cares about the caregivers.*
>
> —Joan Smith, Revere, PA

If you are shaking your head and asking, "Why is she trying to politicize what for me is a very personal undertaking?" please bear with me. There may well be some of you who are still uncomfortable thinking of yourself as a family caregiver, and some of you may find the idea of family caregivers being considered a specific subset of the population disturbing. But that's exactly why I want to share with you some of what I have learned over the years, about how much things have changed in terms of health and healthcare during the past century, and how they are having a very real daily effect on me and my family, and on you and yours.

Healthcare Achievements 1900–2007

All across this country, public personalities and unknown citizens have lived so much longer than anyone would have imagined because of the extraordinary advances that have occurred in medical science and technology.

Christopher Reeve, who was the beloved superman of the movies, died last year, eleven years after sustaining a horseback-riding accident that left him a quadriplegic and turned him into another kind of superman, a man with an inner strength of steel that propelled him to be a spokesperson and fundraiser for spinal cord injury research. If Chris's accident had occurred five years earlier, the medical knowledge, skills, and equipment needed to save and maintain his life most likely would not have been available, and if there had not been continual advances he might not have lived as long as he had, given the severity of his disability.

Also in 1995, on September 15, Kaylee Davis was born with a rare genetic disorder called Kniest Dyplasia. She has heart, lung, orthopedic, and hearing problems, to name just a few. She has required up to fifteen medications a day to survive. The medication must be administered via a *G-tube* that goes directly into her stomach, as does the liquid food that is her diet. She has had more operations in her short life than most of us will ever have in our lifetime. She's had four in the past two years. Without the advances in medical science that have occurred since her birth, Kaylee would not be alive today. In fact, doctors gave her little chance of surviving since most children with her condition die at birth. Lest you think Kaylee's life is only about medical interventions, let me assure you that she is a bright and perky eleven-year-old. She's just completing fifth grade, receives As and the occasional B, and knows how to have fun. This past summer she was a member of a Challenger Baseball Team for children with special needs.

Given the medical wonders of our time, it is easy to forget that in the early 1900s infectious diseases were the most common cause of death. More than 675,000 people died just in the United States alone from the influenza outbreak of 1918. Although it is commonplace today, penicillin was the miracle drug of the early 1940s. A vaccine for polio, the great crippler of children, became available in 1955 and this was soon followed by an oral vaccine in 1963 that was much easier to administer and therefore became accessible to an even larger number of people.

Everyone from the baby boomer generation has a small-pox mark somewhere on their upper arm, a sign that we had been vaccinated against this disfiguring and deadly disease. Early generation Xers, including my daughter, have one too, but not my granddaughter. In 1972 the United States Public Health Service advised against inoculating children for small pox because it was no longer seen as a threat to the American public. We had for all intents and purposes wiped out one of the most infectious diseases in the world.

It was only in 1978 that the first sign of what would later be called *AIDS* showed up in the United States. It shortly became an epidemic and was considered a terminal disease. Although many people still die from AIDS, it has been reclassified from a terminal to a chronic disease because of the many drugs that have been developed in this short period of time to keep the AIDS-causing virus under control. And the research continues. A recent Google search found 57,400 articles about new scientific research findings related to AIDS just between 2002 and today.

One of history's most extraordinary scientific efforts, the charting of the human genome, was begun in 1990. It was completed in 2003, two years ahead of schedule and only fifty years after the discovery of the DNA double helix. These sorts of rapid discoveries are changing the face of medicine on almost a daily basis. Issues surrounding stem cell research are part of the politics of our times, but that wasn't true prior to the 1990s. Dolly, the cloned sheep, was born in 1996. In 2006 the U.S. Food and Drug Administration (FDA) issued a draft risk assessment that found meat and milk from clones of adult cattle, pigs, goats, and their offspring are as safe to eat as food from conventionally bred animals.

If you drew a chart of all the scientific and medical advances since 1900, you would see what is often referred to as a *J-curve*, one that very slowly starts to move, almost laterally at first, and then shoots rapidly and radically upward. Such change in one aspect of our lives has a direct effect on other aspects as well, but that doesn't mean that these changes are absorbed and integrated into society at the same breathtaking speed. In fact, social change always occurs a great deal more slowly.

The Snail's Pace of Social Change

Although we have learned how to save the lives of people who are injured by gunfire or suffer a heart attack, we haven't put in place an organized, affordable, and easy-to-access way for them to learn about and obtain the services and social supports necessary to continue living a meaningful life. Once that survivor leaves the hospital, it is up to her and her family to figure out how they will put bread on the table, pay bills, move easily around the community, and continue to have a network of friends and family willing to help out during a crisis and long into the future.

Doctors can restore a man's health after a stroke, but there is no guarantee that he and his wife will be able to cope with the fact that he can no longer speak or walk as steadily as he did before, and there is no one person, or team of people, for them to call who will jump into the breach when they need help navigating the new and rocky terrain of their daily life. This was made abundantly clear during the recent scandal about the bureaucracy at Walter Reed Army Medical Center. Soldiers returning from the Iraq War were facing significant obstacles in getting the services and disability payments they needed and deserved. If those who have risked their lives aren't being given the services they need and deserve, why should we be surprised that the rest of us are having a hard time getting them?

One of the things that frustrates family caregivers more than others is the fact that they are left on their own to wade through a patchwork sea of disparate programs that may or may not be open to them or meet their needs. Everyone working in the field of caregiving agrees, our system of social supports is hopelessly fragmented and insufficient, and there is no good and easy way to fix it. Family caregivers need the mental acuity and passionate perseverance of a Sherlock Holmes to even solve one part of their support-needs puzzle. I don't know if it will make you feel any better, but even medical and social service professionals have trouble finding what they need when caregiving turns personal. If they can't, why is it assumed that we can?

Kaylee Davis can truly be called a miracle of modern medicine, but it is the hard work and the enduring love of her family that must be forever vigilant to ensure that her life has quality as well as years. Science and medicine may be on a J-curve, a rocket-powered trip of discovery, but the path to implementing the day-to-day rights and services needed by the Kaylee Davises of this world is traveled by well-meaning and dedicated people riding ox carts to reach their destination. This vast difference in the speed of change between science and society is one of the primary reasons that caregiving is, and will continue to be, such a challenge for both caregivers and care receivers unless something can be done to bring them closer together.

I don't mean to suggest that there are no services for family caregivers, but rather that they are hard to find, often have waiting lists, differ from state to state, and are not open to all family caregivers. In the resource section you will find some helpful phone numbers and Web sites to check out.

The Aging of the Population

One of the outcomes of all of these scientific and medical discoveries is the fact that most of us are living longer and healthier lives. We just celebrated my mom's ninetieth birthday on March 1. She's in great health, reads about current affairs voraciously, and leads an active life as a volunteer and grandmother to two generations. She is constantly amazed that she is still alive because both of her parents died at what we would consider today to be quite young ages: her father at fifty-eight and her mother at sixty-seven. They both died from heart attacks suddenly and unexpectedly. Given the fact that they were born in the late 1800s, that's not surprising, but actually both of my maternal grandparents beat the odds. The average life span in 1900 for an American was only forty-seven. Today the average age is seventy-four for men and seventy-nine for women. It has lengthened by about three months every year since the mid-nineteenth century. By the time I was thirteen, all four of my grandparents had died. But my mother has already lived to see her grandchildren marry and become parents themselves. One of my favorite photographs is of my mom, me, my daughter, and her daughter; four generations all alive at the same time. In 1900 only 25 percent of newborns had four living grandparents, and only 2 percent did by the time the child turned fifteen. By comparison, children born in 1976 had a one in six chance of having all four grandparents alive by the time they turned fifteen.

My mom is part of the fastest growing age cohort in the country. According to the Census Bureau, by 2050 there will be 33.7 million people in the United States who will be more than eighty years old but at the beginning of the twentieth century there were only about one thousand people who reached that advanced age. Demographers project that by 2030 there will be more than 380,000 people who are at least one hundred years old. I, and some of you, may well be one of them.

Because so many people are living longer, the definition of old has changed. Researchers now divide the sixty-five and older population into three segments. There are the *young old* (sixty-five to seventy-four), the *old* (seventy-five to eighty-four), and the *oldest-old* (eighty-five and older).

We truly live in an age that is radically different from previous ones, and because of that, the role we are playing as family caregivers is new too. As we have seen there are both positive and negative consequences to the amazing scientific and medical achievements that occurred in the twentieth century and continue today.

Quicker and Sicker

Given the advances in medical science, it is not surprising that the practice of medicine has changed over the years, and it is not surprising that the costs have gone up as well. Just think about the alphabet of high-tech medical tests that have become so familiar to us: EKG, CAT Scan, MRI. Managed care seemed to fall into our lives out of nowhere as an answer to the rising costs of care. It sounded great in theory, but the fact that most consumers would rather be in preferred provider plans that are more flexible suggests that medicine needs to be high quality and consumer friendly as well as cost effective.

The healthcare we knew in our youth is definitely a thing of the past. When laws have to be passed to ensure that women can stay in the hospital for twenty-four hours after they deliver a baby, something is definitely out of whack. If you or your loved one have had cause to be in the hospital recently, you know that the maternity ward isn't the only place that is on a fast track, in-and-out schedule. There is even a term for this quickened pace of discharge. It is referred to as "quicker and sicker."

This is no laughing matter. Just because people are being sent home sooner doesn't mean that they are healing any faster than they did before; it's just that the place where healing occurs has shifted from hospital to home. And that is where family caregivers come in. Families are being asked to do for their loved ones what a team of healthcare workers used to do in the hospital.

Some family caregivers have to monitor the intravenous flow of medications that could previously only have been provided in a hospital setting. Others must learn how to clean and dress serious open wounds that only nurses or doctors were allowed to treat in the past. Feeding tubes, ventilators, catheters, and syringes, you name it, family caregivers are becoming all too familiar with medical equipment and jargon. On the one hand, we are being thrust into the role of healthcare provider. On the other, we are rarely provided the solid training we need to feel comfortable and competent in this role. We learn by trial and error, not on a dummy in a classroom setting under the watchful eye of a professor, but in our own homes on someone we love.

This just doesn't make sense. Doctors don't treat their family members precisely because of the emotional connection. They go through twelve years of education and training before they are considered sufficiently qualified in their area of specialization to be given the full responsibility of a severely ill patient. Nurses too have years of training and must pass a rigorous exam and work in a clinical setting before they are allowed to put RN after their name. Physical and occupational therapists are certified. Nursing assistants are required by federal law to have at least seventy-five hours of training and take an exam before they are certified to work with patients.

Not so for family caregivers. In a series of focus groups held by the United Hospital Fund of New York in 1997, family caregivers talked about how they experienced the hospital discharge process. Their comments were integrated into a groundbreaking report, "Rough Crossings: Family Caregivers' Odysseys through the Health Care System."

Caregivers experienced discharge from the hospital as an abrupt, upsetting event because hospital staff failed to prepare them technically and emotionally for changes in the patient's condition. In many cases, participants reported, after discharge the patient required nursing skills or equipment they did not possess and had little time to acquire.

One caregiver whose husband had had a stroke talked about her concerns regarding the use of a feeding tube with confusing computer settings that she was expected to monitor. "I was terrified of it. . . . It's broken twice. When we left the hospital they showed me one, two, three, and that's it. They said, 'Don't worry, you'll learn it.'"

A man whose wife had MS and underwent surgery for a leg infection thought that at the time of discharge his wife would be in the same shape she had been in upon entering the hospital. He was not told that she was incontinent or that her bandages would need changing. During the first night home when her bandages were oozing and the bed was wet with urine he found out. "I didn't know what to do, who to call, or who to get angry at," he said in total frustration.

These are not isolated statements. In NFCA's 2001 "Survey of Self-identified Family Caregivers" half of the respondents said they had not been given the training they needed. They had to figure things out on their own.

The Two Different Worlds of
Chronic Care and Acute Care

One of the main reasons that all of these outlandish situations exist is because in America we finance, deliver, and provide healthcare in ways that are antithetical to the kind of care so many people need. Our entire healthcare system has always been built on an acute-care model and not a chronic-care model. In reality, what we need is a healthcare system that provides quality care in both domains.

Acute care deals with here-and-now problems that require immediate attention, such as an appendix that needs to come out or a car accident victim who must be operated on immediately in order to stop internal bleeding. In acute-care medicine, cure is always the goal. In chronic care situations, the kind that family caregivers deal with every day, cure is not possible. Chronic-care situations are long-term and are not only medical in nature. They cross the line and require functional assistance such as transportation and personal care. There are psychosocial and environmental issues that must be dealt with, such as the need to build a new self-image after an amputation or figuring out how to make your home wheelchair accessible. The treatment of chronic conditions requires a holistic approach to healthcare, but unfortunately, American doctors are not trained to treat chronic conditions or teach patients and their families how to manage them. This is a growing problem because care of the chronically ill accounts for more than 75 percent of all healthcare expenditures.

It is not only the training of doctors that creates this disconnect between what patients and families need and what healthcare provides. Physicians aren't paid to provide the kind of care needed by the chronically ill. Listen to this 1998 testimony before the Senate Finance Committee given by Dr. Alan Lazaroff, who at the time was Director of Geriatric Medicine and a specialist in chronic-illness care at the Centura Health System in Colorado. Unfortunately Dr. Lazaroff's testimony is just as relevant today as it was back then.

> *Much of my most important work is unrecognized and uncompensated—adjustment of medication, early detection of problems, referrals to and coordination of other services, teaching and counseling. If I hospitalize a patient, I can bill Medicare every day I make a hospital visit, never mind whether this is the most appropriate treatment. If I meet with family members of a patient with Alzheimer's disease, coordinate with other professionals, counsel patients and families about both the benefits and limitations of aggressive treatment, and help my patients cope with the emotional consequences of their illness, I can bill nothing.*

It's clear that American healthcare is out of sync with the reality of life in America today, in which chronic illnesses and family caregiving have the starring roles. Unfortunately despite the fact that there is more research and some action on improving chronic-illness care, the daily lives of most caregiving families have not improved in the five years between the initial publication of this book and today. But there is reason to be hopeful. Researchers and advocates, thought leaders and politicians continue to look for ways to make life better for persons with chronic illnesses or disabilities and their families. It is, at least, a front-of-the-mind issue today, and there have been a few big strides.

Congress passed the Medicare Modernization Act of 2003, which included for the first time Medicare payments for prescription drugs. The program is far from ideal, but millions of Medicare beneficiaries now have better access to prescription medications and this is a good thing. In 2006 Congress passed the Lifespan Respite Care Act to make respite more available and affordable for family caregivers, and reauthorized the National Family Caregiver Support Program. In these ways and more there is a slow trickle of change, but so much more needs to be done before family caregivers can live lives devoid of depression, fear, and financial distress.

Healthcare Insurance: Public and Private

Medicare and Medicaid are the government's two major healthcare financing programs. Medicare is America's answer to healthcare financing for the elderly and disabled, and Medicaid was developed to pay for healthcare services for the poor and disabled. Most people are not enrolled in Medicare or Medicaid but private insurers often take their cues from what Medicare does and does not cover, so the Medicare rules have relevance for all of us. So do the Medicaid rules, because those of us who have a loved one in need of nursing home care usually have to decide whether or not to apply for Medicaid, a decision that has significant financial consequences.

Medicare

Medicare was instituted with fanfare in the 1960s and rightly so. It was the first federal program designed to pay for hospital care and doctors' visits for our senior population. At the time, most seniors were in their sixties and needed treatment for immediate, acute-care problems for a short duration, conditions such as a broken hip or pneumonia. But as we've seen, a great deal has happened since then. A great many of the folks who were in their mid-fifties and mid-sixties when the program began are in their eighties and nineties today. They are suffering from chronic conditions, such as Alzheimer's disease and other dementias, hypertension, diabetes, emphysema, long-term cancers, and the aftermath of a stroke, which they were much less likely to survive in the 1960s. In fact today, more than 300 million people in America are living with at least one chronic condition.

The kind of care today's old and oldest-old seniors need is more extensive than the care they needed forty years ago. It is more long term, and much of it isn't quite medical, although it is necessitated by medical conditions or the frailties that come with old age. Some need help maintaining a household including shopping, paying bills, and housekeeping. Others can't manage these tasks and also are unable to take care of their personal-care needs, such as dressing, toileting, bathing, and other activities of daily living. Between age sixty-five and sixty-nine, only 9 percent of the population requires such help, but within the eighty-five and older population, 50 percent of individuals need such assistance.

Medicare was never designed to pay for the long-term personal care and therapeutic services that people with chronic conditions need. They just aren't part of the Medicare package. In fact, Medicare doesn't even address personal care. It inappropriately, and I think pejoratively, refers to the type of services provided by family caregivers as "custodial care," and as you and I know, what we do is far more than watch over our loved ones, which is how the dictionary defines the word *custodial*. But regardless of what words you use to describe the services family caregivers provide, many people assume that Medicare covers them, and therefore they and their families have a rude awakening when they least expect it.

It's worth taking the time to look at Medicare in more depth, not only because it affects millions of caregiving families, but it is a good example of how "un-caregiver friendly" our healthcare system really is.

Physician Time

Some of the rules and regulations that affect us the most have to do with the privacy rulings under the Health Insurance Portability and Accountability Act (HIPAA). These are not part of Medicare, but it is important to mention them here because some physicians are interpreting the privacy rules to mean they are not allowed to talk to family caregivers, and they are being very adamant about it. If a doctor won't even talk to you, you and your care recipient have a bigger problem than which services the doctor can bill for.

Assuming a doctor is open to talking with you, and even sees you as an ally in his patient's care, there are no CPT codes (the boxes they check on the payment form) that allow a physician to bill for time spent talking with and counseling family caregivers if the patient is not also present. When a doctor is not being paid, there really is only so much time he or she can afford to spend with us. What this regulation is saying in no uncertain terms is that Medicare doesn't recognize the role of family caregivers. This is the crux of some other issues as well.

In addition to not paying for doctors to talk with us, Medicare also does not allow a physician to bill for time spent coordinating a patient's care with other doctors. Given that most care recipients are dealing with multiple physicians, this is a serious issue. Lack of care coordination is believed to lead to unnecessary hospitalizations, and to otherwise unnecessary nursing home stays. It is also thought to be one of the primary reasons for a patient to experience an adverse medication reaction. If your loved one's doctors aren't communicating with each other, how is each to know what the other is prescribing? The answer is that it becomes your job to tell them. By default, family caregivers are the health system's care coordinators.

Yet another problem related to the physician payment rules is that doctors are paid less for taking a patient's history and performing an examination than for performing a procedure, even if the former takes more time than the latter. Yet, time to describe problems adequately and be counseled about symptoms and the pros and cons of potential treatment options is what family caregivers and their loved ones need. Performing an endoscopy or interpreting an MRI might be more lucrative for a physician. These diagnostic procedures are required from time to time, but they don't represent the type of care people with chronic illnesses need daily. It would seem that doctors should receive more money to better care for the chronically ill. It would benefit family caregivers, and our loved ones, to have more time with them.

Definition of Homebound *and Related Issues*

If you haven't come up against the homebound rule you'll think I am making this up; unfortunately, I'm not. Medicare says that unless someone literally can't leave the house without assistance, he or she is not eligible for home-care services. If that individual does leave the house for anything other than a medical reason and this is discovered, the services will be suspended. This was changed slightly some years ago to allow people to go to religious services a few times a month, a graduation, or a funeral, but it has to be clear that these are not everyday events. The home-health services that Medicare will pay for must be considered "medically necessary"—to treat a pressure sore, for example—or be of therapeutic value, and Medicare will only pay for services for a short period of time, not over the long haul. Part of the reason for this, as noted before, is that Medicare was designed as an acute-care system (performing heart surgery, curing ear infections, or saving the life of someone who has been in a car accident, etc.) and has not adjusted to the changing demographics of our society, or the fact that people are now living many years with chronic conditions such as Alzheimer's, the consequences of stroke, and MS. Regardless of the reasons, it leaves caregiving families in the lurch, having to pay out-of-pocket for help with "activities of daily living" such as transfers and toileting.

CMS (the Centers for Medicare and Medicaid Services, the agency that oversees Medicare) is not willing to pay for a power wheelchair for someone to get around outdoors if that person doesn't need it inside the home. Common sense tells us that in a house there are walls to hold on to, the distances are not very vast, and many homes don't have doorways wide enough to accommodate power chairs. Since Medicare provides services for people with disabilities as well as the elderly, this could mean the difference between someone going to work and having to be on welfare. In fact, the disability community is so outraged by this ruling that a coalition was put together just to fight this provision.

Don't get me wrong, Medicare is a wonderful program, but it does need to be overhauled to meet the needs of our time, and the foreseeable future. Here are some more reasons why.

Therapies

Medicare is starting to pay for a few preventive services. In 2005, Medicare began paying part of the costs for a one-time physical for new enrollees, and a blood test every five years to screen for heart disease, but it still does not cover physical therapy, occupational therapy, or other rehabilitation services if it cannot be shown that the patient is improving. Many ill and disabled individuals need these services over a long period of time so they don't lose more ground, to help maintain current functions, or to slow down the impact of a debilitating disease. If your loved one falls and breaks a hip, Medicare will pay for him to go to the hospital and have an operation, but not for therapies aimed at preventing the fall in the first place.

Caregiving Goods and Services

Medicare does not cover basic supplies that are needed by many caregiving families—the most obvious being adult incontinence products. These can easily cost $1,800 annually. Medicare will pay for supplies, however, if someone requires catheterization. Releasing urine from the body with an implement is considered a medical procedure, and therefore it is covered, whereas capturing urine if it just flows uncontrollably from the body is not. Isn't it all about the same thing, controlling urination?

Medicare does not cover any of the costs of home modification to make a house safe for a senior or person with disabilities, such as grab bars in the bathroom or building a ramp at the front door. And perhaps it shouldn't. After all these are not medical expenses. Yet research shows that everyone would much rather stay in their own home than go to an institution. The Supreme Court even ruled in the 1999 Olmstead decision that people should have the ability to live in the "least restrictive setting" possible, which, for most of us, is at home. It would seem that being able to pay for the means to do so and prevent accidents from happening should be part of the bargain.

Another Medicare ruling that is particularly loathsome for family caregivers is the refusal to pay for the cost of a fully electric bed, even if the caregiver's back has already been damaged by bending and lifting and her or his ongoing health is at risk.

Medicaid

Unlike Medicare, Medicaid pays for many long-term care services for people meeting its strict financial guidelines—though the most frequently funded services are those in nursing homes and other long-term care facilities. Whereas Medicare is administered by the federal government, Medicaid is not. Many of the program's services vary from state to state, but all states must pay the cost of care in a nursing home or other institutional setting for those who qualify. Legislation has been proposed to actually give Medicaid beneficiaries control over an individual budget for personal care and related services—often referred to as the "Cash and Counseling" model. Generally, however, Medicaid funding goes directly to service providers and beneficiaries do not have much of a say in how it is spent.

In the initial Cash and Counseling demonstration projects that were conducted in three states (Florida, Arkansas, and

New Jersey), money was provided directly to Medicaid recipients to determine (within reason) how they wanted to spend it. These demonstrations have proven very successful. In some cases, people decided to pay a family member to provide their care services. This program is now being expanded, and twelve additional states are in the process of implementing Cash and Counseling programs. A related concept is the "Money Follows the Person" program, which is also being expanded. It provides funding for individuals to move from nursing homes to community-based settings, and is something for family caregivers to watch. Aging and Disability Resource Centers (ADRC) are being developed on the state level to create a single, coordinated system of information and access for all persons seeking long-term support. The goal is to minimize confusion, enhance individual choice, and support informed decision making. Currently, forty-three states have received grants to create an ADRC. The idea is to provide "one-stop shopping," so regardless of which state you live in you can call a central number to find the answers to your questions. The idea is a great one and it is exciting to see this beginning. It will take a while for many programs to become fully operational before we know if the programs will truly have resources and programs specifically for family caregivers or only for their care recipients. Making sure they do would be a good activity for someone who wants to get involved and help make life better for family caregivers in their state.

Nursing home care costs average $57,000 a year, and can be twice as much in major metropolitan areas or in hard to reach places. In Alaska for instance the average cost is $167,000 annually. Most of us can't come up with that kind of money. Since Medicaid was specifically designed for low-income individuals and families who do not have insurance or resources to pay for their healthcare, middle-income people have truly been caught in the middle with Medicare not providing long-term care services at all and Medicaid only providing it for a strictly defined population. To make the situation more equitable for the middle class, Congress established rules for long-term care that allow individuals to "spend down," which is a euphemistic way of saying deplete, their assets and thereby qualify for assistance. It used to be that when a two-person household was involved, for example a husband and wife living together, this "spend down" practice left the well spouse (often referred to as the community spouse) in poverty without enough income or assets to cover his or her own basic needs. According to changes to the 2007 Medicaid guidelines, spawned by the efforts of advocates for the elderly, community spouses are allowed to maintain between $1,650 and $2,541 a month of income, and between $20,328 and $101,640 in assets, as well as their house, car, and other personal effects and still be eligible for payment of nursing home fees. Because Medicaid is administered at the state level, actual numbers vary across the country.

> *I took care of my 91-year-old mother and my disabled sister. Think how much money my 6 ½ years of caregiving saved the system in nursing home fees.*
> —Judy Sing, MaComb, OH

Workplace-based Health Insurance

Most family caregivers who are neither eligible for Medicare or Medicaid get health insurance coverage through their employers. Large employers, because of their strong buying power, can usually negotiate significant savings and more benefits for their employees than smaller ones. Some employers cover the full cost of health insurance for their employees but the number is steadily declining as the cost of healthcare takes up a bigger percentage of a company's costs. Other employers pay a partial amount and as healthcare premiums go up, as they are doing now, employees are being asked to pay more and more of the premium out of their own pocket. Self-employed individuals often have to find creative ways to obtain reasonably priced health insurance, and some people, such as those who work part-time (many moms of children with special needs fit into this category), may not even have the option of employee-offered benefits, and therefore must find a way to pay for individual policies or decide to go without coverage at all.

Caregivers who received their health insurance through their loved one's employer prior to his becoming ill or disabled and having to quit the workforce know the devastating impact that loss of health insurance can have. The entire family is left up the proverbial river to fend for itself in the rising-cost waters of non-employer based policies. Even if the caregiver can subsequently obtain coverage from her employer, her loved one, because of his now preexisting condition, may be caught without any insurance at all. Family caregivers themselves who stop working in order to meet their caregiving responsibilities are in the exact same boat when it comes to finding a new, affordable policy.

When preparing to give testimony before the Senate Subcommittee on Oversight of Government Management Restructuring and the District of Columbia in the summer of 2001 on the health insurance issues facing the caregiving community, I sent a query to a random selection of caregivers on the NFCA email list asking them to share their thoughts and experiences regarding health insurance. Some people were just thrilled that I even brought up the subject since it is so little talked about. Others sent in very poignant accounts of what has happened to them and their families and I included a number of them in my testimony. These comments are typical.

> *I quit work to care for my husband and paid an exorbitant amount for COBRA insurance for both of us. When that ran out, I had to get an individual policy (which he was not eligible for) and pay for it myself.*
> —Janet Miesiak, Allen Park, MI

> *I have been caregiver for my mother and aunt, both in their 80s, since 1991. I had to quit my job last year when my mother had another heart attack. I lost health,*

dental, vision, and disability insurance, plus pension and deferred compensation. I am presently retaining my health insurance through COBRA, but it costs me $304 per month and it will run out.
                              —Sandra Jacobson, Bellevue, WA

Family Caregivers Are Literally Underpinning Our Healthcare System

As you've read, there are many consequences of being a family caregiver in America today. None of us as individuals can address them alone but by pooling our individual voices we can bring our concerns to the attention of local communities, states, and the federal government. Then, and only then, will caregiving families have a chance at a quality of life that is comparable to that of the non-caregiving majority of Americans.

Family caregivers provide more than 80 percent of all long-term care services. The market value of the services provided by family caregivers was estimated to be $306 billion dollars in 2004, a 19 percent increase over the previous estimates made only four years earlier. Family caregivers are literally underpinning our healthcare system and are an irreplaceable resource. Virtually all of the country's functionally disabled seniors receive some of their care from family caregivers, and almost two-thirds receive all of their care from family or friends. As you would expect, children with special needs predominately get their care from one or both parents.

I think the economic benefit that family caregivers provide is underestimated. Before I took over the care of my parents, they were in the doctor's office at least once a week.
                              —Wendy Wharton, Oak View, CA

Family Caregivers Put Their Own Health at Risk, Sometimes in Dramatic Ways

Family caregivers are known to have a much higher incidence of depression than the rest of the population, six times as much for spouses providing thirty-six hours of care a week or more and twice as high for the adult child of aging parents who provides that level of care. Some studies have shown that depression among family caregivers lasts longer than the depression experienced by patients. In fact, family caregivers of Alzheimer's patients continue to experience stress up to three years after their loved one has died. Family caregivers often suffer from significant sleep disorders and back problems. Medical studies have shown that the stress of caregiving can cause caregivers' immune systems to function more slowly and thereby increase wound-healing time. Other medical studies have shown that elderly caregivers under extreme stress have almost a two-thirds higher mortality rate than non-caregivers and caregivers who don't experience significant stress. We even age more rapidly than non-caregivers, another study showed, up to ten years more quickly. Family caregivers don't need statistics to tell them about the physical and emotional impacts of caregiving. They have their own experiences.

Stephanie was born with one quarter of one kidney. Although most new moms don't get a lot of sleep, I virtually got none because of her interventions and reactions to medication. After three months I had lost twenty pounds, had terrible bags under my eyes, and looked like a zombie. The doctor threatened to hospitalize me because I was suffering from exhaustion. When I started thinking it would be a nice break I knew I was in trouble.

—Lauren Agoratus, Mercerville, NJ

It's Expensive to Be a Caregiving Family

I spend $600 to $800 on homecare aide services every month and that's because I was able to find a non-certified aide who works for me directly. It would cost me more than twice as much if I went through an agency. I have a friend who is paying over $1,000 a

month because she needs an aide for more hours than I do.
> —Evie Rosen, Edwards, CO

Families in which one member has a disability spend two and half times more on out-of-pocket medical expenses than non-caregiving families, more than 11 percent of their income. This is not surprising when you consider the cost of products and services such as diapers for school-age children and incontinent adults, installation of grab bars, accessible vans, respite care, and personal attendant aides.

[My wish is] to have the legislature mandate that health insurance companies cover the expense of incontinent supplies. In our case, the yearly cost is $1,500 to $1,800.
> —Sheue Yann Cheng, Potomac, MD

Covering these costs is even harder when a family's income has been reduced because either the caregiver or care receiver has become a part-time employee, turned down a promotion, or left the workforce entirely. When that happens, not only is income reduced, but so are potential future pension benefits and social security payments. Caregivers are very often put in an untenable financial position and may not even realize the full impact of it until they themselves need care. It is not surprising that a higher percentage of caregiving families live in poverty than their non-caregiving counterparts. Financial concerns are worrisome for most caregiving families, but seem to be worst for parents of children with special needs, many of whom are now living on into adulthood and even old age. Who is going to be able to support or supplement the income of these adults with special needs when their parents are no longer alive?

Caregivers at Work

Not only are the repercussions of caregiving affecting families in their personal lives, they are also having a profound effect on them in the workplace. Companies both large and small are trying to find ways to keep productivity up while simultaneously giving employees the flexibility they need to care for their ill or disabled loved ones.

The majority of family caregivers, 59 percent, are employed outside the home, and 62 percent have had to make some adjustments in their work life. Businesses are very concerned about the growing number of people involved in caregiving and rightly so. They are losing billions of dollars a year, as much as 33.3 billion, because of it. Some of the cost is caused by increased absenteeism, reduced productivity on the job, and the costs associated with replacing workers who quit. Approximately 25 percent of U.S. businesses have at least some information and referral services to help family caregivers meet their familial responsibilities and still be productive workers. Ironically though, only about 2 percent of caregivers at these companies take advantage of the programs that are available to them for a variety of reasons. Some simply don't believe that they should bring their personal lives to work; others are concerned that by telling their manager about their personal situation, they may jeopardize their jobs. There is some evidence to support this concern. In her column on work and family issues for the *Wall Street Journal* of September 13, 2000, Sue Shellenbarger wrote:

> *Many readers who responded to a recent column on workplace discrimination against caregivers to the elderly and disabled had their own stories of being treated badly at work because of caregiving duties.*
>
> *Among about 50 readers who responded, several said they had to lie to gain the flexibility they needed. Others were forced to quit their jobs.*

There is no question that our personal lives affect our work lives. Win-win solutions for employees and employers must be found. Traditional programs to support family caregivers in the workplace consist of providing access to information, but today there are some pretty creative solutions being tried out that go way beyond that.

Case in point, Fannie Mae the country's largest non-bank financial services company (which basically means they help make it possible for many people to buy a home), has a very innovative family-caregiver support program going back as far as the late nineties, and it came about when Fannie Mae's then-CEO, Frank Raines, proposed hiring a geriatric-care manager to help employees solve problems related to family caregiving and elder-care issues. Mr. Raines realized that Fannie Mae needed to go beyond the flexible scheduling, telecommuting, job sharing, and part-time opportunities that were already in place. Caregivers needed someone who knew the ropes to actually locate resources and help them make decisions.

This corporate commitment to providing employees with real assistance in finding solutions to their caregiving problems is good business. Other companies, such as Prudential Insurance, are paying for subsidized emergency backup care. The company has found that it prevents absenteeism and workday interruptions. Verizon offers a similar service and Raytheon provides in-home assessments and care planning. Wouldn't it be nice if more companies followed these models? Workplace problems would be one less thing that family caregivers needed to be concerned about.

Caregiving in the Legislative and Public Policy Arena

The title of this book is *A Family Caregiver Speaks Up: It Doesn't Have to Be This Hard* and "It Doesn't Have to Be This Hard" is also the title of this chapter. I firmly believe that public policy directly affects what happens in the bedrooms and bathrooms of caregiving families. I and the board of the National Family Caregivers Association believe this so strongly that removing the barriers to family caregivers' health and wellbeing is an essential part of the organization's mission. It is encouraging that family caregiving and its consequences are of much greater concern to Congress and state legislatures than they were five years ago, when this book was first published.

As we all know, until somebody experiences family caregiving, they can't fully comprehend its difficulties. More and more of our elected officials are beginning to experience caregiving first hand—and it is turning on light bulbs. In fact, in the summer of 2006, a handful of advocates for family caregivers and/or the elderly and I were called to a meeting by the then-chairman of the House Energy and Commerce committee, Joe Barton (R-TX). Much of the legislation that affects family caregivers goes through this committee and, thus, Mr. Barton had considerable influence and power. A close family member of the Congressman's had been diagnosed with Alzheimer's disease and he was seeing its effects. The purpose of the meeting was to discuss legislation to help family caregivers that could possibly be passed before the Congressional session ended. No legislation actually came out of the meeting, nevertheless the meeting was historic and clearly illustrates that the reality of what it means to be a family caregiver is being felt in Congress. Now, more than any time in the past, family caregivers have a chance to be heard and have a say in legislation that affects us and our loved ones.

The first piece of national legislation to recognize the role of families in providing care was the Family and Medical Leave Act (FMLA), passed in 1993. The FMLA allows an employee, in an organization with more than fifty employees, to take twelve weeks of unpaid leave from work because of their own health needs or the health needs of a family member and still retain their job. Since its enactment, the FMLA has helped more than 50 million employees deal with significant healthcare situations without having to worry about potential consequences at work. Research by the National Partnership, the organization behind the FMLA, has shown that many more people would take advantage of this opportunity but they can't afford to give up their paycheck during the time they'd be at home. The National Partnership is actively working to find ways for employees to be compensated during their time off and to expand the benefits to employees at smaller companies. At the same time it is fighting back the possibility of limits to the law. In the meantime, California became the first state to offer paid medical leave in 2004 and others states are looking into the possibility as well.

California has always been ahead of the curve when it comes to supporting family caregivers. In 1980, the state authorized a pilot project to provide services for family caregivers of persons with Alzheimer's disease. Four years later, the statewide system of eleven resources centers was formed. They provide a wide range of services to family caregivers including assessment, counseling, respite, and consultation on care planning, legal matters, and more. California is the only state in the country with such a comprehensive program.

Other states such as New Jersey, Pennsylvania, Wisconsin, Washington, Oregon, and New York were early adopters of innovative programs, too. You can find out what public programs exist in your state by visiting www.caregiver.org, the Web site of the Family Caregiver Alliance.

States have been ahead of Congress in other ways as well. Oregon, Wisconsin, Nebraska, and most recently Arizona implemented legislation that established statewide, lifespan-respite programs. In these states, lifespan respite provides a coordinated system of accessible, community-based respite-care services for caregivers regardless of age, race, ethnicity, special need, or situation. Other states, such as Oklahoma, have implemented similar programs without legislation, while still others, such as Maryland, have put in place the mechanisms needed for building local systems to assist caregivers in accessing lifespan-respite programs. Congress has finally caught up and, as the 2006 congressional year ended, it passed the National Lifespan Respite Care Act. It took more than four years and the work of many individuals and organizations to get the bill passed. Changing policy is not an activity for those with little patience. But this is a democracy and therefore citizens, including family caregivers, can, have, and must continue to speak up for their rights.

The year 2000 was a very exciting year for family caregivers. That's when Congress passed, and then President Clinton signed into law, the National Family Caregivers Support Program (NFCSP). This was the very first piece of national legislation to specifically provide for support services for family caregivers. It called for the establishment of programs, administered through Area Agencies on Aging, to provide support, information and referral, decision-support training, respite to family caregivers, and, in some instances, direct services. The program was approved for five years and then the legislation would have to be "reauthorized" if it were to continue. Through the efforts of NFCA and many others the National Family Caregiver Support Program was recently reauthorized for an additional five years.

I can hear some of you saying, "That's nice. I haven't benefited from any of this." Neither have I. I don't work for a large company and NFCSP focuses on the neediest amongst us. Steven and I don't fit into that category. That isn't the point though. Legislation is never universal. It always targets specific populations, but once a bill is enacted into law, it provides a precedent for further legislation that can expand the reach of the program to additional portions of the population.

Every year bills that would help family caregivers are introduced in the House of Representatives and/or the Senate. Many of them don't have a chance to become law because of political or budgetary reasons, but the fact that they are introduced represents a stake in the ground in support of caregiving families. There are actually a significant number of bills already introduced this year that would have a positive impact on the lives of caregiving families. They include a tax credit for family caregivers, social security credits for those leaving the work force to care for a loved one, care coordination services for Medicare beneficiaries who have multiple chronic conditions, and more.

In the 110th Congress, which is the congressional session that began in January 2007, fourteen bills that would have an effect on family caregivers were introduced in the first half of the year. For example Sen. Edward Kennedy (D-MA) and Rep. Rosa DeLauro (D-CT) introduced the Healthy Families Act. This bill provides paid sick leave to employees "to ensure that Americans can address their own health needs and the health needs of their families." Specifically, the act mandates that employers with at least fifteen employees provide a minimum paid sick leave of seven days annually for employees who work at least thirty hours per week, as well as a prorated amount for those who work twenty to thirty hours per week. It allows employees to use the leave to meet their own *or* their families' medical needs.

Sen. Susan Collins (R-ME) introduced a wide-ranging healthcare bill whose provisions include: tax credits to small businesses so they can provide health insurance for their employees, tax credits to individuals when buying health insurance, deductions for the purchase of long-term care insurance, and tax credits for individuals with long-term care needs (care recipients). A list of the bills introduced in Congress between January and June 2007 that would have an impact on family caregivers and their loved ones, if they were enacted into law, can be found in the appendix.

These and other actions on the state and national level all point to a growing awareness of the needs of family caregivers and their loved ones and the realization that, although caregiving is an issue that families deal with on a very personal level, society needs to support family caregivers and address the consequences of their role on a community and governmental level. For the promise of past initiatives to turn into expanded and on-going programs in the future, family caregivers need to become involved in the debate and speak up for what they and their loved ones need. In a representative democracy such as ours, the stories and voices of constituents make a very real difference and are often the reason some pieces of legislation actually get passed.

A family caregiver who participated in an NFCA-sponsored focus group some years ago commented:

I don't think being a caregiver is a political statement
where I have rights. . . . It sounds like you're being an
advocate for something. It just takes all the softness and
the love out of it.

She couldn't have been more wrong. You do have rights and by standing up for them you are expressing great love for your care recipient because your wellbeing and their wellbeing are intertwined. Family caregiving is hard and always will be, but it doesn't have to be as hard as it is. You may not be able to cure your loved one's condition, but together we can cure the public policy ills that make living with it so much harder.

My Personal Vision of a
Family-Caregiver-Friendly America

Do you believe the negative consequences of caregiving are fair? Do you believe that love and responsibility should be penalized rather than rewarded? I don't.

Do you think that Medicare and Medicaid, as well as more businesses, need to be caregiver friendly and that additional caregiver-friendly legislation should be enacted at the state and federal level? I definitely do.

I think caregiving families handling significant medical issues should have access to a care-coordination team to help them adjust to crises and changing situations and make sure that correct patient information is transferred from doctor to doctor and from hospital to rehab to home. I think a Medicare payment system needs to be established to reflect the reality of our lives and the needs of the chronically ill as well as those with acute conditions. I think family caregivers should have input into the design of community-based programs aimed at helping them and their loved ones, and that medical education needs to be reformed so that doctors have a greater understanding of how to work constructively with the chronically ill and their family caregivers. I think many things need to be done to create a more level playing field for caregiving families as they confront the game of life.

I know that life isn't fair. We are all dealt a hand at birth and events intercede in both wonderful and horrific ways. I also know that the negative consequences of family caregiving were never intended and have come about because of a confluence of discoveries and circumstances. All the more reason that we should strive to reduce the negative impact of caregiving on individuals, families, and society. In fact, now that we are aware of the inequities, we must try to correct them, not only for our own sakes, but also for all of the family caregivers who will follow us.

In 2003, NFCA and a number of other organizations and individuals that care about helping family caregivers through the legislative process got together and developed "Family Caregiving and Public Policy: Principles for Change," a document to provide guidance to legislators. NFCA publicly presented the principles at a national town hall meeting on Capitol Hill early in 2004 and they still form the basis for caregiver-friendly legislation today. There are eight principles in all. These are the first three.

- Family caregiving concerns must be a central component of health care, long-term care, and social service policymaking.
- Family caregivers must be protected against the financial, physical, and emotional consequences of caregiving that can put their own health and wellbeing in jeopardy.
- Family caregivers must have access to affordable, readily available, high quality respite care as a key component of the supportive services network.

All of the principles are in the appendix. Some of the members of the original group, including NFCA, have recently banded together to create the Family Caregiver Public Policy Work Group with the goal of proposing (and getting passed) Medicare and Medicaid legislation that will benefit family caregivers. If we succeed it will be a great milestone.

Currently neither program addresses our needs. Neither program even recognizes them.

There's a Way for Everyone to Be Involved

I suspect many of you are saying, "I don't even have time to take a relaxing bath in peace; how do you expect me to get involved in changing the world?" I don't. I'm only asking that you start to think about helping to make life better for your loved one and yourself. That's really not any different than what I suggest throughout this entire book. I'm just asking you to think about it in a slightly different way than you usually do.

It is important that you acknowledge your role as a family caregiver. What I mean is that it is important to recognize that our love and sense of responsibility, our ethics, our marriage vows, and the very fact that we are parents compel us to care for our chronically ill, disabled, or aged family member, partner, or good friend. The job of family caregiving often demands an excessively high price that far exceeds what a just and compassionate society should ask of its citizens.

A Step All Family Caregivers Can Take: Acknowledging Your Role

Moving from the concept that caregiving is strictly a personal issue, something not really to be talked about in public, to the belief that family caregivers are part of a very large and ever-growing constituency that deserves recognition by others does not require time or energy-draining action. It does, however, require thought and consideration of the information laid out in this book. If you can do that, if you can acknowledge to yourself that you are a family caregiver, you will already be making a difference. Research has shown that family caregivers who self-identify as caregivers are more proactive in support of their loved one, more confident in talking with their loved one's doctor, more apt to be concerned about their own welfare, somewhat less isolated, and definitely more cognizant of the connection between their personal caregiving and broader social issues. The very act of self-identifying can increase your ability to be a more effective and healthier caregiver and a more proactive person who speaks up for the rights of family caregivers.

How to Get Involved, One Step at a Time

If you do have some time and energy to spare, if you are sufficiently upset about the current state of affairs that caregiving families find themselves in, you can move beyond acknowledgement to action.

You can try to read more articles or listen with more attention to the TV news when healthcare issues are being discussed. By being better informed you are making a difference. You can discuss what you've read or heard with others and draw examples from your own experience. That way you are putting a human face, a face the person you are talking to actually knows, on the statistics and issues in the news, and thereby getting others to see them through a different lens, a more personal and compassionate one, that might make them talk about these issues to more people, and so the chain grows.

If you are part of a support group, you can suggest that the group talk about a specific topic of concern, such as paid family leave or social security benefits for non-working family caregivers. The members of the group can gather data, come to conclusions, and write a letter to your state or federal representative, either individually or collectively.

You can agree to share your story with the media so that the general public can gain a clearer picture of what caregivers lives are really like. You can try to be part of a local community or even a state coalition, advising officials on caregiver-related issues.

You can become part of the NFCA community (there is no charge for family caregivers), lessen your loneliness, gain practical knowledge through our print and online newsletters, and stay on top of the public policy debate. You can add your story to the hundreds of others we've collected, find a pen pal, communicate with other family caregivers and be part of our ever-growing community. You can support NFCA's efforts to assist caregivers now while simultaneously working to bring about social and legislative changes to make your life easier. As the strength of our collective voice grows, so does the possibility of change.

You can do one or more of these things depending on your time and your inclination. Each one will make a difference. It all starts with believing that family caregiving goes beyond you and me, that it is a personal issue, but also very much a societal one. Will you stand up and be counted as one of the whole, one family caregiver among millions, who believes, "It Doesn't Have to Be This Hard"?

For those interested in the differences between advocacy and action, I recommend "Advocacy and Activism: Missing Pieces in the Quest to Improve End-of-Life Care," an article by my friend Ira Byock, a noted doctor who is a leader in the palliative-care movement.

> *Advocacy by individuals can directly improve care for a patient. However, organized public participation, or activism, is required to alter institutional and professional policies, curricula and standards of care. The individuals who are involved in activism may be patients and their families. However, patient and family involvement is activism rather than advocacy if improving care for groups of patients, or systems of care, is a goal.*

Sometimes actions can have both advocacy and activism as concomitant goals. The time is right for family caregiver advocacy and activism. As Helen Keller noted: "if we all do a little it will add up to a whole lot."

CHAPTER 4

Building Confidence and Capabilities: Making Choices, Taking Charge

YOU are the only person who can take charge of YOUR life.
—Jane Hedrick, Jenks, OK

Often people become caregivers suddenly, without warning. Your husband was diagnosed with cancer and requires extensive chemotherapy. Your teenage son had a car accident and is brain injured, unable to think clearly and respond appropriately. Your mother had a stroke that left her without use of her right side.

At other times, caregiving creeps up on you. You know dad is forgetting things, and you slowly start taking on some administrative tasks and calling more often, until one day you realize he no longer has the capacity to live safely on his own.

Regardless of how you became a caregiver, whether it was a terrible shock or somehow slipped up on you, in the "hubbub" of the day-to-day routine, amidst the reorientation of your schedule, the search for resources, and the fears about the future, you probably never stopped to think about exactly what happened. You probably didn't devise a plan to help you deal with the present situation or look ahead to what the future had in store. If you are like most family caregivers, you just went into autopilot and started to do, and do, and do.

Somewhere along the line, however, it is vitally important that you stop, take a breath, and try to gain some control over the situation, rather than letting the situation control you. It is vitally important that you choose to take charge of your life.

> *If you don't [take charge of your life], you will become bitter and resentful, and your self-esteem will ultimately suffer. You will lose sight of the reason you chose to become a caregiver in the first place, which is because you love that person and want what's best for them.*
> —Kim Barrett, Port Orange, FL

What does that mean—choose to take charge of your life? Obviously you cannot control everything that happens to you or to your loved one. If you could you would make their illness or disability go away. You would banish caregiving from your life and bask in the heady air of health, wellness, and "normalcy." But even though you don't have that power, you do have the power to make active choices about how you are going to deal with the caregiving circumstances of your life.

Attitude

> *Everything negative has a positive side. Keep on looking until you find it.*
> —Betty S. Katz, Deerfield Beach, FL

> *A caregiver cannot take charge. The loved one's condition changes. . . . You can merely co-exist, maintain some sense of self, and plan for better days.*
> —Martha Harnit, Eustis, FL

Perhaps the most important choice you have to make is how you are going to approach life from here on out. You can choose to drink the sour and acidic juice of lemons, or you can try to make lemonade out of them. You can view life as a glass that is half empty or one that is half full, and if you choose the latter view you will inevitably be a happier and healthier person. You will also be a more peaceful and loving caregiver, and more capable of proactive action on behalf of yourself and the person you care about and for.

That's because attitude impacts action. Our inner thoughts propel our outward movement. If you put on the mask of self-pity, then you'll shoot a hole in every idea or suggestion that well-meaning people offer. If you wallow in the waters of negativity, you just may drown. I know. I wallowed for a very long time and I paid the price in multiple ways.

> *Just fake it! Act as if . . . then it makes it easier to be cheerful. Soon, you will actually feel positive. It's a decision, not a feeling.*
> —Nancy James, Odessa, TX

I'm not suggesting that you be a Pollyanna. That doesn't make any sense either. Complete denial of your changed situation has as many negative side effects as wearing a hair shirt. What I am suggesting is that you recognize that you do have choices. There may be more difficult choices now that you are a family caregiver and have a loved one dependent on you in ways you never imagined. It is also true that some of life's options that were once open may now be closed to you and your family, but life still offers options and choices, and recognizing that will help you have a life that is rich and good and full, albeit in different ways than it was before. So much depends on our attitude.

Evie, the friend I mentioned before, is the perfect example of a family caregiver who revels in life and always finds its silver lining. She refers to herself as a realistic optimist. She says:

> *I have always believed that all the information we need and want is out there in the universe. But it doesn't*

just appear. You have to believe it is there and make the
effort to find it. You have to believe that flowers can
grow from rocky soil.

I must admit I'm not like Evie. At times I tend to see the negative side of situations first. I can't immediately see the good that comes out of the bad, the rainbow after the downpour. That's why it is so good to have a friend like Evie. She can always help me see things through a brighter lens.

A positive attitude requires constant attention and
practice.

—Judy Black, Portland, OR

How do you view your glass, as half empty or half full? Caregiving may bring forth a common grab bag of emotions, but how we deal with them is very individual and reflects our attitude toward life in general.

A year after Cindy and I went on our respite to the beach we were fortunate enough to have the opportunity to go again, but at the last minute she had to cancel, so I went by myself. It wasn't an easy decision to make, but I'm glad I did. I needed to do some thinking and soul searching, and this gave me the opportunity.

It was a rather sad time for Steven and me because he had recently gotten his first wheelchair, the scooter no longer being sufficient for his needs. Although the wheelchair definitely made our day-to-day life easier, it was a symbol of his growing disability. It caused the old emotional wound that started with the diagnosis to reopen, and so once again I had to confront my fears about disability and our future, my sadness and my pain, and Steven had to confront his as well.

While at the beach, sitting on the sand and soaking up the warm rays of the sun, alone with my thoughts and feelings, I wrote a poem that was inspired by, of all things, a beach chair. The poem erupted out of my brain in only a few minutes and poured onto the writing pad that was propped up against my thighs. It was a very dark poem, reflecting all the painful emotions the purchase of the wheelchair engendered. It expressed my fears and my anger. It was the visible representation of the pain that I held inside. It was a poem written by a woman who definitely saw her glass as half empty. The sun was shining. I was enjoying a respite, and I decided to try to think about Steven's need for the wheelchair in a different way. I ripped up the first poem and began again. The poem that came from my inner core the second time around was more upbeat. It looked at the doors that the wheelchair opened for Steven and me, not the ones that it had closed. This is the poem I called "The Chair," but wonder now if I should rename it "Life Depends on Your Point of View."

It sits there at the crest of the beach, on the rise just before the sand dips towards the water's edge.
A lone beach chair, seemingly abandoned.

It's a jaunty chair with its yellow striped canvas seat and sailboats floating on its blue and yellow back support.
It lists just a bit to the left, almost rakishly, as it nestles in the sand, surveying the sea.

It is a chair made just for sitting, and sitting on the sand at that. It has no legs to get in the way of stretching out, relaxing, and letting the sun seep into your bones and warm your soul.

It is so unlike another chair I know. A black chair with wheels. A chair that does not survey the vastness of the ocean with a jaunty air, but rather a chair that defines a narrower kingdom.

And yet, I think this other chair is a happier chair than the one that sits and stares out to sea, for it is a chair with wheels that take the place of legs no longer able to propel their owner forth.

This other chair is not made for sitting and looking at the world. It is a chair built for exploring, for meeting life face to face and tasting of its spirit.

Perhaps this chair should have a seat of yellow and white stripes, and a back support adorned with sailboats.

A far better statement of its adventurous and joyous possibilities.

Nothing had changed in the hour between the time I wrote the first poem and the time I wrote the second one, nothing except my attitude. And yet that was everything.

Take Charge Activities and Coping Strategies

It's a fallacy to believe that we are ever in complete control of our lives. So much happens because of situations well beyond our ability to affect them; yet they affect us, sometimes for the good and sometimes for the bad. A big rise in the stock market can mean you'll definitely have enough money to send your kids to college. A tornado can destroy your home beyond repair. Other circumstances we obviously do have some control over. We can choose where to go on a vacation or choose to put ourselves on a low-salt diet to control high blood pressure. A loved one's illness or disability generally falls into the first category, and we struggle to find ways to control its impact on their life, on our own, and on the lives of the rest of the family. We need to find ways to regain some of the sense of control that we've lost. We need to learn how to cope.

A Personal SWOT Analysis

Have you ever heard of a SWOT analysis? It is something that is done in the business world to assess a company or an organization's ability to change or move forward. It is often one of the first steps in strategic planning. SWOT stands for strengths, weaknesses, opportunities, and threats. To get a handle on your life as a family caregiver, to begin to take charge, to find ways to cope with your fears, to determine what choices you have, you might consider conducting your own personal SWOT analysis.

We all have strengths and weaknesses. These are characteristics that are intrinsic to who we are. Some of them may be physical, some intellectual, some an innate part of our personalities. They may change over time, or a perceived strength may be an asset in one situation and a liability in another.

Have you ever thought about your strengths and weaknesses in terms of your caregiving situation? If you haven't done it yet, you might consider making two lists. List number one can enumerate what you see as your strengths and what impact each one has, or could have, on your ability to be a successful family caregiver. List number two includes your perceived weaknesses and the consequences they have, or could have, on your caregiving. These lists can help you sort out in which areas you could really use some assistance or advice.

In my case, I'd say one of my strengths is the fact that I tend to be proactive and plan ahead. I can also be persuasive. I can laugh at myself. I usually catch onto things fairly quickly. I don't have a problem asking for help, and I am physically stronger now than I have ever been in my life.

In terms of weaknesses, I am a five-foot, small-boned woman, and although Steven is an average-size man, I just don't have the leverage to help him if he falls or needs other significant physical assistance that requires height. I am lousy with math. My eyes glaze over when it comes to filling out forms, and I can be impatient, especially when dealing with bureaucracy.

Opportunities and threats come from the outside. A retirement community is being built two miles from your house, or your husband's employer will let him work from home two days a week. These are obviously opportunities that, in the right circumstances, could be the answer to your prayers. Threats can range from a potential loss of health insurance to the fact that you live in an old two-story house that would require extensive, and expensive, renovation to make handicap accessible.

Can you think of what opportunities you currently can take advantage of, or what threats you need to find ways to work around or somehow get rid of? A personal SWOT analysis is a place to begin to think about questions such as these, and it is one of the arrows in your quiver of resources to help you build your confidence and take charge of your life. Think of it as a living document, one that will change as you and your circumstances do. It can be a useful tool throughout your caregiving career, not just at the outset.

Being Proactive versus Reactive

Knowing more about yourself and the circumstances that could have an immediate effect on your situation is a start, but taking charge of your life shouldn't end there. Over and beyond gaining an understanding of what you bring to your caregiving situation, there are other actions you can take to boost your confidence and give you more of a sense of ease. It is important to remember that, although you can't control everything that happens, you do have the power to choose your responses and whether you are going to let circumstances take control of you, or you are going to take control of circumstances.

I strongly believe that family caregivers need to become strong advocates for their loved ones and themselves, and that we need to be proactive and resourceful in finding the information and help that we need. Having said that, I also recognize how difficult it is for already over burdened caregivers to find the energy and wherewithal to battle unresponsive healthcare and social-services systems, and unfortunately, sometimes other family members as well, and to meet their loved one's needs, especially if being a fighter doesn't come naturally.

I also know that many of you will do just that. You will find an inner strength you didn't know you had and you will make an effort—indeed, are making an effort every day—to resolve yet another problem with the insurance company, put the pieces in place that will allow you to get away for a day of respite, track down the cardiologist and get him to coordinate with your loved one's primary care doctor. It's hard to be an advocate for yourself and your loved one, but if you or someone you delegate to are not, then life will be that much more difficult because caregiving doesn't come easily, and the services and supports we need unfortunately aren't part of a seamless whole.

Being an advocate means recognizing that you and your loved ones are consumers and, as consumers of our healthcare system, are owed quality care, respect, and responsiveness. Being an advocate means recognizing that the squeaky wheel is often the only one that gets attention in a too-busy system. Being an advocate means fighting for what you believe is right—whether that is an extra day in the hospital or a timely report on a new set of tests. It's getting your boss to understand that now you need some time off, but that you have a plan in place for meeting your responsibilities to the company, and being an advocate is also about getting at least one other family member to recognize that now and then you are going to need a break and they are going to have to chip in with hands-on care.

The dictionary defines *advocate* as both a noun and a verb. As a verb it means, "pleading on behalf of something or someone." A suggested synonym is the word *support*. That being the case, you may have long been an advocate without even realizing it.

Parents know that it is important "to pick your battles" so that you aren't arguing with your kids all of the time, and so that when you put your foot down they know that you mean it. Another way of expressing the same thing is to say, "Don't sweat the small stuff." All of this is good advice for family caregivers who have to conserve their energy and decide what's worth making a fuss over and fighting for. But just recognizing what is important enough to expend your energy on is a big step and a positive advocacy approach.

How are you going to be proactive? How are you going to be an advocate for your loved one and yourself? There are many possible ways. For instance, are you going to educate yourself about your loved one's condition and your rights as a healthcare consumer so you can play a real role as a member of the healthcare team, or are you going to accept the information provided to you as gospel without asking questions or trying to insert yourself into the healthcare process?

Are you going to be proactive and do some planning, such as obtaining a medical power of attorney so there will be no question of your authority to speak for your loved one if he can't speak for himself? Are you going to learn skills that will make caregiving a safer process for you and your loved one? There are a variety of ways you can build your confidence and capabilities, but you first need to choose to take charge of your life. Research, planning, and skill development are just three of the ways to develop your confidence and capabilities. Don't assume you have to do all of these simultaneously or all by yourself. Part of the process of taking charge is prioritizing and coming up with a game plan. Your SWOT analysis can play a role.

Research Takes Many Forms

Not knowing is being lost.
                    —Rhonda Huffman, Toledo, OH

For many people anticipating becoming family caregivers or those newly thrown into it, one of the first things they want to do is learn about their loved one's condition. Having a base of knowledge about his diagnosis can put you in a better position to ask the doctor meaningful questions about treatments, side effects, and prognosis, and also help you better evaluate recommendations given. Do you know some of the common terminology associated with your loved one's condition? What research could you do to increase your knowledge base and, with it, your confidence?

One place to go for information is a voluntary health agency (VHA); that is the general term for organizations like the American Heart Association, Easter Seals, and the Brain Injury Association. VHAs focus primarily on finding a cure or treatments for the particular illness or condition they represent, but depending on their size and their mission many provide all sorts of services to help patients cope with their diagnosis and its impact. In the past few years, some VHAs have begun to recognize that their sphere of concern needs to include family caregivers as well as patients, and consequently your research may turn up information and programs specifically designed to help you cope with, and become more capable at, the job of family caregiver. In the resource section there is a list of many VHAs, their Web sites, and their toll-free phone numbers.

The Internet is the place of choice to do research these days. You can read articles written for the professional community, chat with others in similar circumstances, post questions for a doctor, create a medical journal for your loved one, stay up on the latest legislative activities that impact services for those with physical and mental disabilities, and have a conference with other members of your family. The list of what you can find out and what you can do on the Internet is seemingly endless. Information is empowering and, generally speaking, the more you have the better off you are. I'm definitely not an Internet whiz kid. Nevertheless when I want and need to know something about MS, I get online and search away. I now know the addresses of some specific MS sites, but at the beginning I just went to a search engine and typed in MS. A list of sites to look at popped up. If you are just getting started, that's what I would suggest you do. Don't have access to the Internet? I bet someone you know does and they'd be happy to help out in this way.

> *The internet has been my lifeline to the information I need.*
> —Janet L. Kieffer, Mingo Junction, OH

Some years back, when Steven started having difficulty urinating and a visit to the doctor suggested this was probably a long-term problem, I immediately turned to the Internet to learn more about his condition. We were very aware that incontinence is a big problem for many people with MS, but we'd never heard of anyone who suffered from urine retention. It never entered our heads that MS could cause someone to be unable to pee. After a couple of hours in front of the computer, I surely wasn't an expert on the issue, but I knew enough to talk intelligently to the urologist and to ask reasonable questions. I even happened on a research article he wasn't aware of. Talk about a sense of confidence, let me tell you. When I faxed that article to him I felt so much more capable as an advocate and a family caregiver. And it was amazing how differently the doctor began to treat me. I wasn't just Steven's wife anymore; I was an important player in the discussion and decision-making process who was to be taken quite seriously.

Learning as much as you can about your loved one's condition is a critical activity that isn't only important at the beginning of your caregiving journey but one that continues throughout it.

> *Research is a mixed bag. Obviously I read everything I can get my hands on . . . and sometimes I feel more in control. Other times, it just highlights what might be in the future and I don't always want to think about it.*
> —Anita Bluestone, Teaneck, NJ

> *Research has been a big help in helping us to understand the tests that are being done and what to expect next. It helps us to make more informed decisions and feel that we still have some control over our lives and decisions.*
> —Linda C. Jackson, Norman, OK

Rules of the Game

There's another kind of research that is equally important to do if you want to feel more in command of your caregiving life. It's finding out the rules of the game. What I mean by that is the world of healthcare is complex. It has its own systems of operation designed to help the medical personnel involved do their jobs, prevent injury, and maintain proper records. These systems are not designed to accommodate families.

For instance, it is important to understand that a doctor's legal responsibility is to the patient, not to you the family caregiver, unless of course you hold medical power of attorney. If you and your loved one want you to be part of the decision-making process, want you to be present during examinations and tests, then it is your loved one who must communicate that to the doctor, assuming she is mentally and physically able.

Just as the medical profession as a whole has its rules, so do physicians' offices. And just as with other businesses, rules differ from one to another. A good way to find out how a doctor's office works is to get to know the office staff. Learn people's names. It goes a long way toward creating a relationship as opposed to just an exchange of information. The office manager or nurse can tell you the best time of day to reach the doctor by phone, what days and hours the office tends to be busiest, what procedures must be followed if you need a prescription refill, and even the lead time involved if you want to make an appointment for a routine exam. If you know how the office is run, you are much more likely to avoid frustrating situations.

The same is true in emergency rooms and when someone is admitted to the hospital. There are procedures, and in some cases actual rules, that must be followed there too. For instance in the ER, especially if it really is a dire emergency, your job is to provide necessary information quickly and then get out of the way. In the hospital, one thing I have found is that providing a typed list or computer form of Steven's critical information is immensely helpful for the medical personnel I have to interact with. It's helpful for me too. I try to update it periodically and always take a copy of it and Steven's living will and power of healthcare attorney with us on any hospital visit. You may have heard the term *personal electronic health record* (PEHR) or *personal health record* (PHR). These are records that are "owned" by the patient. You and your loved one are the only people who connect across all healthcare settings: doctors' offices, hospital, rehab, home. Therefore you are the only ones who can provide a complete record of your loved one's history and status. The field is still in its infancy and at this point I find it easier to use a typed form that includes core information about Steven's condition and his functional abilities. You can read more about personal health records in the article in the appendix.

Medical Information Form for Steven Mintz	
Name and Address:	Steven Mintz
Home Phone:	XXX-XXX-XXXX
Insurance:	Company and Policy Number
Medical Issues:	Mr. Mintz has Multiple Sclerosis.
	He requires urinary catheterization.
	He has no other medical conditions, but there is a history of diabetes in his family.
	He has no known allergies or adverse reactions to medications.
	Both his father and mother are deceased. (Dad heart, mom cancer.)
Blood Type:	O Positive
Care Issues:	Mr. Mintz is in a wheelchair. He requires help with all activities of daily living.

Care Issues (con't.):	He cannot transfer on his own. To get him onto a hospital bed or gurney, two people are needed, one to pick him up under his arms and the other to lift him beneath the knees.
	Mr. Mintz's fine-motor skills are greatly impaired. It is best to assume that he cannot manipulate anything on his own, except perhaps the emergency buzzer.
	Our experience is that after a hospital stay, Mr. Mintz is temporarily more disabled than he was at admission. Home-care assistance is definitely needed to help him with ADLs.
Doctors Names and Phone Numbers:	
Primary:	XXXXX/XXX-XXX-XXXX
Specialists:	XXXXX/XXX-XXX-XXXX
On-going Medication:	Name, amount, dosage, special instructions (e.g. Lipitor, 10 mg, once a day, in the evening)
Call in an Emergency:	Suzanne Mintz
Relationship:	Wife
Phone numbers:	Work, Home, Cell
Documents:	Mr. Mintz has a Living Will. Mr. Mintz has a Medical Power of Attorney designating Mrs. Mintz as his surrogate when necessary.

Note the detail under "Care Issues." You'd be surprised how little doctors, and even nurses understand about the limits of people with disabilities, which are compounded when they are ill.

Being prepared to work within the system, or being aware of what you will face if you try to buck it, is important information to have so that you are on a level playing field with the professionals with whom you need to interact. There's nothing more unnerving or confidence deflating than to believe you are the only actor in a drama who hasn't seen the script, and if you think about it, that is exactly your situation in healthcare settings. Everyone you will meet has been trained and, in most cases, licensed or certified to do their job. They are familiar with the procedures and rules. You and your care recipient are the only ones working in the dark. That being the case, the more questions you can ask, the more organized you can be, and the more you act like a healthcare advocate, the more confidence and control you will have over your caregiving circumstance. Information on planning a doctor's office visit and other practical tips on interacting with the healthcare system can be found in the appendix.

Peer Knowledge

> *By doing research, I also have found other people willing to share their specific experiences, and I know that I am not alone. I have found that I am also able to help other people by sharing the knowledge that I have acquired.*
>
> —Judy Horner, Boardman, OH

Some of the best research you can do involves talking to other family caregivers. Learning from those who are somewhat farther along in their journey than you and your loved one, or have actually completed it, can save you countless hours of effort and provide you with very concrete and practical advice.

There are many products and services available to help caregiving families but most of us don't know what they all are or where to find them, and there's no one place to go that has all the answers. Developing friendships with other family caregivers, caregiving families, or people with disabilities can enhance your ability to find what you need.

My friend Joan isn't a family caregiver. She is a person with a disability and she lives on her own. Joan has a very bad case of rheumatoid arthritis. She has had to revamp her entire life because of her illness and therefore she has searched out and found many products to help make her life easier. Although her illness is very different than Steven's, they have some of the same problems. Joan has a hard time picking up a glass because her fingers are so curled and inflexible. Steven has a hard time picking up a glass because his hands are weak, his fingers are no longer nimble and he has little sensation in them. Joan told us about these extra long straws that she uses. They can be easily cut to whatever length necessary to meet your particular needs. She gave Steven one to try and told us how to get them if we were interested. We find them so helpful that we even keep some in the backpack that we take with us whenever we go out. These straws provide a very simple solution to what is actually a rather big problem, but we never would have known they existed if it wasn't for Joan. Sure, we may have come upon them if we went on a search for a product to help Steven drink from a glass more easily, but we hadn't yet begun to do that, and how much nicer to have a product be recommended by a friend who already knows that it works.

If the shoe were on the other foot, if we knew about the straws and thought they might be beneficial to Joan, we would have told her about them. When we find a superior product or service, Steven and I jump at the chance to share our finding with others. It's part of the unspoken bond that those of us outside the norm make to help each other maintain as much normalcy and independence as possible. So don't hesitate for a second to ask other caregivers or someone you might know who has a disability if they know a physical therapist they swear by, or if they know of a product that makes it easier for a person with limited mobility to get in and out of a car. It might just save you a lot of time, and effort, and anguish.

Doing research, all kinds of research, is definitely one of the ways you can begin to gain some control over your caregiving situation and improve your own sense of confidence and competency in the bargain. If research isn't your forte, if it seems beyond you regardless of the medium being used, or if you just don't have the time, is there someone else in your family, or is there a friend or colleague, or a member of your congregation who can do it for you? Don't think you have to do everything yourself. Learning to be a manager, to delegate tasks, can help you feel more in control. Thinking of alternatives when roadblocks are put up in front of you is yet another way to begin to take charge of your life. It is a proactive approach to problem solving.

Planning

If you have a plan, you can enjoy what you have at the moment without as many distracting fears about the future.
— Victoria Kellerman, Parkville, MD

Since becoming a family caregiver, have you done any financial or legal planning, or even sought advice about these issues? Have you evaluated your finances to see if there is any way you can afford to pay for even a little bit of help? Have you tried to find out if your family is eligible for free or low-cost services through local, state, or national programs? Does your loved one have a will and a living will? Do you? Do you know what Medicare does and does not cover, or, if your care recipient is under sixty-five, what your private insurance will pay for? Are you aware of what might happen as your sister's condition deteriorates, and have you at least thought about what that might mean in terms of her ability to continue living on her own? Have you considered the possibility that you could have an accident or get sick? I know we never think anything is going to happen to us, but what if it did? I wear a family caregiver medical ID that tells emergency personnel that I care for my husband Steven and he will need help. It has given me such a sense of peace and also empowerment I never would have believed possible. Information on medical IDs for family caregivers can be found on the last page of this book. It is amazing how many questions arise when you begin to think "what if."

I am positioning myself professionally to be able to work from home and earn the same, if not more income, if it should become necessary.
　　　　—T. Mikki Crawford, Silver Spring, MD

If anything should happen to me, what happens to my husband?
　　　　—Sonia J. F. East, Copper Hill, VA

I had dinner with a colleague from out of town who was moving to the DC area. Chuck confided to me that his wife had a degenerative brain disorder that was currently affecting her mobility and fine motor skills, so it was important to him to find a house that was either all on one level, or at a minimum had the master bedroom and bathroom on the entry floor. He wasn't sure if his wife would ever lose her ability to climb stairs, but he thought it foolhardy to look for a home that wouldn't be able to easily accommodate his wife's long-term needs. Chuck was being realistic about the future that he and his wife could possibly face, and he was taking that potential future into account when making a long-term housing investment. He was planning, not that she would definitely be unable to walk, but for "what if."

As Chuck told me this, it brought back memories of when Steven and I went looking for our current home. It was in 1987 and although Steven definitely had mobility problems he was still able to negotiate stairs. Despite that, we did exactly what Chuck and his wife did. We thought it a realistic possibility that Steven wouldn't be able to climb stairs at some point in the future and so we only looked at one-story homes. In fact, we went on our search with a very specific accessibility checklist in hand. It included a shower stall in the master bedroom, easy access to the backyard and a garage that had, or could have, an automatic garage-door opener. The house we bought didn't meet all the criteria on our checklist, but it met most of them. Over the years we made some changes to accommodate Steven's growing disability, and although some of them required a bit of ingenuity they were all doable, because of the basic properties of the house we bought. By 2003, however we were looking at a major renovation if we wanted to stay in the house. Our typical five-by-eight bathrooms were just too small to accommodate the realities of power wheelchairs and decreased dexterity.

None of us can plan for all of life's possibilities, but we can definitely plan for some of them. I know from experience how emotionally difficult it is to look ahead toward what your caregiving might entail in the future. Nevertheless, it is very prudent to do some forecasting because if you don't, your life may well be filled with many more crises than it needs to be. Being part of a caregiving family is hard enough as it is. There's no point in making it harder than it has to be. Planning for the future can help put you in the driver's seat of life and also help ward off situations that make you feel dependent.

> *At each step we have tried to anticipate the next problem dad would be facing. . . . In talking with dad's doctor about what to expect, we were plugged into hospice early. . . . This forward thinking has helped us not have to scramble and has helped us be mentally prepared as changes occurred.*
> —Lois Finnan, Newburgh, IN

It's been said that Americans are the only people on the face of the earth who think death is negotiable. I don't know if that's true, but I do know that we have a very hard time talking about death and therefore planning for it. That's the one thing we can, and should, all do, even if caregiving wasn't part of our lives.

Some years ago I had the wonderful opportunity to play a leading role in an extraordinary public education campaign to change the way Americans think about, and deal with, end-of-life issues. The program, Last Acts, was a multimillion-dollar effort funded by the Robert Wood Johnson Foundation, one of our nation's leading philanthropic organizations focused on healthcare issues.

Last Acts created a quiet revolution that changed the way physicians manage pain. It raised the public's awareness of end-of-life issues by working with Hollywood producers to include end-of-life scenarios in major TV shows, such as *ER*. And it taught us that death is a natural part of life that we can and should plan for, and that although it is not pleasant, a family can experience it in a calm and loving way.

You may think this is morbid, but in fact it is one of the most life-affirming things you can do. What a great gift to allow someone you love to end their life on their own terms. We only need to think of the Terri Schiavo case to recall what can happen when your wishes are not known and documented.

Caregiving Skills

I have learned to insert/remove the catheter to remove blood clots and relieve my father's pain quickly. I no longer have to call the doctor or take him to the hospital for this.

—Jane Hedrick, Jenks, OH

In addition to research and planning, there are other things you can do to feel more secure and capable in your actions and therefore more in charge of your life. You can learn some specific skills that help you be a more capable and confident family caregiver. For instance, you can learn how to communicate more effectively with healthcare professionals, over and beyond knowing the terminology associated with your loved one's diagnosis. You may want to learn a few nursing techniques and skills that make tasks easier for you and your loved one or some of the basic skills that physical therapists, special needs teachers, and other professionals go to school to learn and get licensed to do. When we realize everything we need to learn to be comfortable and confident in our caregiving roles, it's no wonder that we so often feel out of our bailiwick. Half of the caregivers in an NFCA survey of family caregivers said they hadn't been properly trained to do the caregiving work they were currently doing, so you certainly aren't alone if you are feeling unprepared.

> *I have become proficient with the laws and rights of the disabled community and make it a point to inform others.*
> —Cynthia J. Cavallaro, Swampscott, MA

There isn't one magic place to go to learn skills that can help you in your caregiving. Some hospitals do provide training programs, so it is worth checking with the ones in your community. If your loved one is eligible for homecare services, the agency providing those can certainly teach you skills and techniques as well. Make sure you know what your insurance will and will not cover. Some policies allow a set number of visits by an occupational therapist or physical therapist if ordered by a doctor, and these professionals can teach you transfer techniques and other life skills. Don't forget the Voluntary Health Agency focused on your loved one's condition. The Red Cross even has an entire curriculum on family-caregiver skills training.

> *I went to my local college and became a licensed nursing assistant.*
> —Janet L. Kieffer, Mingo Junction, OH

Managing Instead of Doing

Research has shown that men approach caregiving differently than women. Whereas women tend to jump in headfirst and do everything themselves, men tend to take more of a managerial approach and delegate or purchase outside services. Regardless of whether you are a man or a woman, you can learn how to manage your caregiving responsibilities as opposed to letting them manage you. A professional geriatric care manager may be able to help you do just that and actually assist you in finding the right solution to meet your loved one's needs and your own as well. Whether your loved one is elderly or not, consider learning some care management skills. Here are some tips from the professionals.

1. Educate yourself on the nature of the disease or disability you're dealing with. Understanding what is happening to your care recipient will make you better able to judge the kind of resources you'll need.

2. Write down your observations and evaluations of your care recipient's strengths and deficits. This assessment will not only help you come to a realistic view of the situation; it will be a handy baseline reference to chart the progression of symptoms and changes. It's also not a bad idea to write down your own strengths and deficits so you can be realistic about your own need for help and support.

3. Hold a family conference and decide who will handle what chores if more than one family member is involved. Making sure everyone knows his or her responsibilities keeps misunderstandings to a minimum and saves one person from bearing the brunt of all the work. Note family meetings work best when there is a third party there to facilitate them. It could be a care manager, or member of the clergy, a long-standing family counselor, or anyone that can be trusted

not to "take sides" and also has the skills to keep the meeting on topic, on schedule, and all parties feeling safe so they can truly say what is on their minds.

4. Keep good records of emergency numbers, daily medications, special diets, back-up people, and other pertinent information relating to the care of your loved one. Update as necessary. This record will be invaluable if something happens to you.

5. Research services in your area, including respite care, adult daycare, nursing facilities, volunteer programs, and churches. Look at them from a dual viewpoint: which ones are there to help your care recipient; which ones exist to help you or both of you.

6. Join a support group or find another caregiver with whom to converse or correspond. In addition to emotional support, you'll be likely to pick up practical tips.

7. Start advance planning for difficult decisions that may lie ahead before you will have to make them. It's much tougher to think decisions through when and if the situation turns desperate. Don't neglect to discuss wills, advance directives, and powers of attorney. These instruments give care recipients the opportunity to make their wishes known, but they can be signed only when a care recipient is competent, so it's best not to delay.

8. Develop your own support system. Be willing to tell others what you need and to accept their help. Other people could easily do some of the research that all of these steps entail.

9. Establish a family regimen. When things are difficult to begin with, keeping a straightforward daily

routine can be a stabilizer, especially for people who find change upsetting and confusing.

10. Approach some of your hardest caregiving duties like a professional. Instead of seeing yourself as a spouse or child, step back and try to insulate yourself from the sense of loss such duties remind you of, concentrating instead on the practical aspects of getting the job done as efficiently as possible. Sometimes your best defense is to distance yourself a bit so you can accomplish the difficult tasks without allowing them to take a constant emotional toll. We all have an image of what our role is as a spouse or a daughter. When caregiving enters a relationship, stress is created because your image of your role doesn't mesh with your caregiving responsibilities. Finding a resolution to these disconnects can ease the situation for everyone involved.

These are just a few of the ways you can begin to take charge of your life now that you are a family caregiver. It's all about incremental steps and small things that make a difference. But remember, small steps over time can add up to big accomplishments and a significantly different sense of self-esteem and capability. Together these two personal strengths can help you feel more on top of things, especially if you can keep your cup of attitude at least half full.

Caregiving Is About Love, Honor, Value—and You

It's about protecting your physical, emotional, and financial health. Rabbi Hillel, one of the great sages of Judaism, is the author of my favorite quote. He said:

If I am not for myself, who will be for me?
If I am only for myself, what am I?
And if not now, when?

I know of course that Rabbi Hillel, who lived at the time of Jesus, wasn't thinking about those of us who are family caregivers today, but when I first read those lines, it seemed to me that his words transcended time and took on new meanings for each age, and that for our age, he was sending a message to family caregivers.

So often we are not for ourselves. On the contrary, we give and give and give to help another. No wonder non-caregivers often refer to us as saints or angels. We have no problem living up to the implications of Hillel's second question.

It is his first question that we have a hard time taking to heart. We tell ourselves we need to get more exercise and more sleep, and we need to find more opportunities to relax or take a respite break. Hillel's first question causes many caregivers to laugh and say, "Yeah, right. I'm going to drop everything now and meet my friends for a cup of coffee, go for a long bike ride, or make plans to get away this weekend."

The rabbi's words can actually be a wake-up call for all family caregivers, if we allow ourselves to recognize that self-care isn't a luxury but rather a necessity that can actually improve our ability to provide high-quality care for our loved one. They can serve as a reminder that loving yourself is not selfish, but rather is a way of honoring and valuing the wonder of a human life—yours.

The Gift of Good Health

Why is it that sometimes acting in your own behalf is so valuable not only for yourself, but also for your loved one? The answer is actually quite simple. If something happens to you, if you get sick, become depressed, can't continue to function as a caregiver at a high level, what then will happen to the person you love and care for? Is there someone ready, willing, and able to jump in at a moment's notice and fill your place? I doubt it. What if you actually died? It could happen. Your own good health must be preserved if you are going to go the distance as a family caregiver. Your own good health is the best present you can give your loved one, and yourself.

A study published in 1999 in the *Journal of the American Medical Association* reported on a study of elderly spousal caregivers. The researchers found that those caregivers who experienced significant stress were sixty-three times more likely to die within a four-year period than non-caregivers and also more likely to die than caregivers in less stressful situations. More recent studies, one with parents of children with special needs and another with spouses whose ill loved one was hospitalized, have also shown premature aging for the parents, as much as ten years' worth, and increased potential for death among the spouses, all owing to the severe stress of family caregiving.

Other studies over the years have also documented the physical and mental repercussions of family caregiving. Depression, sleeplessness, and backaches are commonplace among family caregivers who help their loved one with personal-care activities. One study published in the English medical journal, *The Lancet*, in the mid-90s, described how family caregivers can actually have slower healing times than non-caregivers, the stress having a direct effect on the body's own ability to repair itself. And a study published just a few years ago in the very prestigious *Proceedings of the National Academy of Sciences* showed that caregiver stress can impact the immune system for up to three years after caregiving for a person with dementia ends, thus increasing the caregiver's own chances of developing a chronic illness.

These are extraordinary statements. They are scary. They imply that in certain circumstances family caregivers are literally putting their lives on the line to provide quality care to someone they love. Instead of one patient, we end up with two. Just think about the dire consequences if you were bedridden for a while. Caregivers who let their own health suffer, thinking that their time is better spent caring for a loved one, are actually taking a huge risk. If you are in the hospital suffering from exhaustion, if you neglect a minor cough and it develops into pneumonia, or if you are in a serious car accident, who will be the caregiver? Who would even know that you are a family caregiver? Protecting your health by loving, honoring, and valuing yourself, isn't just a nice thing to do if you have the time. It's essential.

> *Recently one of my daughter's physicians told me, "The worst thing that can happen to your daughter is not her health problems; the worst thing that can happen to your daughter is not having you to care for her." This confirmed and encouraged my attitude as a caregiver that my well-being is my daughter's well-being.*
> —Linda Reid, Oneonta, AL

That's why every time you get on an airplane and the cabin crew recites their safety messages they always end with "if the cabin loses pressure, and you are traveling with a small child or someone else who needs assistance, put your own mask on first." Why is that such an important message? Why are we advised to help ourselves first? It is because if we are gasping for air, how can we possibly assist someone else? The little time it takes to ensure we are breathing normally pays a large dividend to our loved one. It gives us the capability to help them now, and it just may be the critical reason why we can continue to help them in the future.

Imagine you are driving down the highway and your fuel gauge is beginning to look rather low. Eventually the warning light comes on to tell you it is definitely time to fill up. Almost instinctively you start looking for the next rest stop. It's the prudent thing to do rather than taking the chance of getting stuck.

Now imagine that you are that car and you have noticed the warning signs that suggest you need to refuel. You are more impatient than usual and you anger more quickly. You aren't sleeping well and your back hurts constantly. These symptoms are our equivalent of the car's fuel gauge. So why don't family caregivers usually honor those symptoms and recognize it is definitely time to pull over and fill up their own tank?

There are any number of answers to that question, not the least of which is most of us have been brought up on the American ethic of independence. We think taking a break means we are not fulfilling our obligations to those we love, that prioritizing our need for regular exercise and a solid night's sleep implies that we are selfish. After all, a parent's job is to protect and care for their child. Society directs us to honor our parents. Wedding vows are promises made and kept. "For better or for worse" translates for some into being there twenty-four hours a day, no questions asked.

Caregiving Is About Relationships

We forget that all of these dictums imply the existence of a relationship, a relationship between at least two people, and as in all relationships, the views and needs of all parties must be taken into account if the relationship is going to be a successful one. Although family caregivers and care receivers are separate and distinct people, we are linked together in a unique way. After all, family caregivers do not exist unless someone they love needs care. And if that person should die then the family caregiver relinquishes her title.

It is this dichotomy between being an individual and being part of a relationship that is often at the core of a great deal of conflict between family caregivers and care receivers. I believe the conflict often stems from the fact that neither we, nor our loved one, recognize and come to terms with the special quality of this relationship. It is as if we family caregivers and our loved ones are conjoined twins with our own heads and our own hearts, but we are joined at the hip, and by necessity must continuously make accommodations for each other if we are going to live in harmony and accomplish things.

If your care recipient's condition is strictly physical, then it is easy to see why and how two points of view are part and parcel of the caregiving equation. But if your care recipient is developmentally delayed, mentally ill, or brain injured there are obviously extenuating circumstances that change the balance of accommodation and decision making, but they don't change the fact that at least two people are affected by whatever decisions are made, your care recipient and you.

Caregiving is by definition a relationship in which one person needs care and another is called on to provide it. It is about loss and challenges and finding a new balance. It's about recognizing that although one person's health and ability to function independently were the catalysts for making yours a caregiving family, everyone in the family, including you, the primary caregiver, has been deeply affected. A successful caregiving relationship requires that caregiver and receiver recognize each other's needs and rights and feelings that have to be considered, honored, and addressed in an equitable way. And although yours may be the primary relationship, it is important to recognize the impact on other close family members as well, especially children, whether they be siblings, friends, or grandchildren of the person needing care.

*The way I cope best with my caregiving situation is to
have enriching activities that I take part in apart from
my spouse. This is extremely important for me and our
relationship.*

—Anita Bluestone, Teaneck, NJ

I wish Steven and I had understood that back in 1974
when he was diagnosed with MS. It might have saved us a
great deal of pain. We didn't understand how vitally important it was to look at the impact of his illness through each
other's eyes. We do that now. In fact it has become the guiding light of our marriage and how we cope with the fact that
ours is a caregiving family.

Our problem was we couldn't communicate about MS.
We couldn't start a real dialogue about our fears, our sadness,
our different ways of coping. I'm by nature a talker and a
planner. Steven keeps things to himself and prefers to deal
with things as they arise.

Steven is the one with the clinical diagnosis of MS, but
we both are living with it. I wanted to be prepared for whatever might lay ahead. He wanted to continue living as much
as possible as we always had. It was this inability to recognize
that we both needed very different things in order to function successfully with the MS in our lives that led to our separations.

What got us back together and has kept us together now
for more than twenty years was the realization that we needed
to find a way to satisfy both of our competing grieving and
coping styles. What got us back together and has kept us together was the recognition that, although he is the one with
clinical MS, we, the family Mintz, also have MS, at least in a
psychosocial sense, and Steven's needs must be met, but so
must mine.

I have come to understand that he needs time to deal
with his own private hell, with the changes in his body, with
decisions brought about not in the normal course of life, but
because of the MS. I have come to recognize that Steven is a

"quiet fighter" and that for him acknowledging the changes in his body means accepting that there is no turning back to a higher level of functioning. Acknowledging that he needs more help is an acceptance that the MS is taking its toll. It is not an easy thing to do and it needs to be done, not in resignation, but consciously and with dignity, and in his own way.

Simultaneously, the reason he can now more easily acknowledge that my point of view is also valid is because he has come to see his MS through my eyes. He's come to understand that my suggestions to look into a new piece of equipment or ask others for help is not meant to take away his independence but rather to protect his safety and to actually give us back some of the independence that his increasing disability is constantly taking away from us. He's come to understand that I have rights when it comes to how we deal with the disability in our lives, and that, indeed, for our relationship to work and to grow, we both need to give a little in order to gain a lot.

We both learned our lessons the hard way, but that is all in the past. We are stronger for the pain, and our relationship is now constructed on solid ground. This process of viewing situations through each other's eyes is based on love and respect and honoring the fact that Steven's illness is our illness, that we are both affected by it, but need to deal with it in different ways and along a different time continuum. It recognizes that in a relationship, a good relationship, all parties count and everyone's point of view has value.

Permission to Say "No"

Another way to love, honor, and value yourself is to recognize that even though you are a family caregiver, you don't always have to say yes to requests or demands. On the contrary, it is important to acknowledge that you don't have to discard the word *no* from your vocabulary to continue to be a loving and thoughtful caregiver who provides high quality care to their loved one. "Yes, I can and will do this, but I'm sorry, I just can't do that" are perfectly legitimate statements to make. This may sound like heresy. How can I possibly say no, you may be thinking. How can I not continue to give and give when she needs me, when the doctor says these are the tasks that must be done? The reason is because saying "no" now could in the long run provide you with the ability to say, "yes, I can" for a long time to come. It can help you find the balance you need between self-care and caregiving. Family caregivers don't have formal rights enacted by law (at least not yet, but we are working on it) or even established by custom, but we all have the right, indeed the natural instinct, to self-preservation.

When doctors or other health professionals assume that you can do specific tasks or therapies or be at the hospital at a specific time to take your loved one home, they generally have no idea what your other obligations are, and unless you set them straight they will go on assuming that you can and are willing to do whatever they ask, when they ask it.

> *It all comes down to setting boundaries.*
> —Lauren Agoratus, Mercerville, NJ

Anne Montgomery, a forthright health policy analyst I know, told me how she stood up to a doctor when he gave her a list of instructions for caring for her dad who had just had heart surgery, after he was released from the hospital. She said,

> *I told him in no uncertain terms that I had other responsibilities. I could not be at the hospital the next day to take my dad home, and I could not stay with him in his house while he was recuperating, that he [the doctor] needed to order some homecare services for my dad. He was assuming that I had no constraints on my time. He didn't consider whether I had a job or a family. When I told him he couldn't make those assumptions, and he realized I wasn't going to kowtow to him, he came up with another plan that was much more reasonable. He let my dad stay in the hospital an extra*

*day so I could make arrangements to pick him up and
wrote an order for homecare services so that an aide
would come in every other day for a week to give him a
bath and help with some other personal needs.*

Not everyone has Anne's gumption, but at times we
would all benefit if we did. A strong sense of self and a belief
in what is right and wrong with our healthcare system has
become a necessity for all of us who want to have some control over our loved one's wellbeing and our own, rather than
allowing standard practice and assumptions of the medical
community to add to the stress of our lives rather than ameliorate it. We already know healthcare in the United States is
not designed to meet the needs of those with chronic conditions or disabilities. All the more reason to develop the confidence to push back when you and your loved one are not
getting the information and service you need.

Recognizing the need to say no, to demand answers to
questions, is one thing; training yourself to do it is quite another. It goes against everything we have been taught about
how to behave with healthcare professionals and against our
natural instincts on how to help those we love, but if we are
going to maintain our ability to provide care for an extended
period of time, we need to learn some skills and techniques to
help us be more effective advocates for our loved ones, and
ourselves, especially when dealing with hospitals or healthcare
professionals.

It's important to remember in caregiving change is a
constant. The lifting you could easily do three years ago may
be having dire consequences for your back today. The sleep-
less nights you were able to rebound from in your thirties
may be a serious health risk in your fifties. By honoring the
rhythms of your body and your mind you are honoring your
own life and the contributions you make to your loved one's
wellbeing.

It takes a lot of courage to admit you aren't superwoman
or superman and that you can't carry on the way you have

been. When it comes to caregiving, it takes a lot of courage and determination to say no and choose another path, even if only temporarily. Maybe that's why less than 30 percent of the respondents in a 2001 NFCA survey of self-identified family caregivers said they strongly agreed with the statements, "I feel comfortable saying no when asked to do more than I think I can by professionals" and, "I feel comfortable saying no when asked to do more than I think I can by my loved one." Learning to say no when it comes to our loved one's requests or doctors' orders doesn't come easily. It is something we have to practice over time and then know when it is the appropriate response.

I know how hard it is because I've said no to Steven from time to time. I recall one time when my doctor told me I was suffering from fatigue and anxiety. She gave me some medication to help me sleep through the night, something I hadn't done for months. I decided getting enough sleep needed to be my number one priority if I was going to be able to function successfully. And I decided that returning to a regular pattern of exercise, another "good for me" endeavor that had fallen by the wayside of caregiving, would be my number two priority.

Unfortunately in order for me to do both of these things, Steven had to alter his nighttime schedule. Steven likes to stay up until at least eleven on weeknights, and even later on weekends. I like to be in bed no later than 10:30 p.m. and at times even earlier. He is also more comfortable going to sleep on his back and then being shifted onto his side four or five hours later. I decided I couldn't do that all the time anymore. I said,

> *No, I need to try and get as much uninterrupted sleep as possible. I need to wake up refreshed and try to get some quality exercise at least three mornings a week. I need to take care of myself as well as of you. Because I have to help you undress and get into bed, I need you to honor my needs more than your own*

*for a little while. In the long run we need to find an
equitable compromise.*

The most recent time I yelled "stop" was just a couple of
years ago when I actually experienced "burn out" for the first
time. Our lives had been even more stressful than usual for
more than a year partially because of our home renovation
project we undertook to make it possible for us to "age in
place," as the current terminology goes. To do this we had to
move out for six months, which is a story in itself. It was just
after we returned that all of the emotion of our experience,
and the impact of the added effort and energy required on
my part, came crashing down around my ears. I remember
shouting at Steven, "I can't do this anymore. I don't want to
do it anymore. We need to find some help." As you can imagine having someone other than me provide some of the personal-care services that Steven requires was a big decision for
him emotionally, and for the both of us financially. Now that
help is in place though, I know it was one of the best decisions we ever made. We hired a wonderful young man who
sleeps over twice a week and helps Steven get into bed, and
assists him during the night if necessary, and then gets him
up, showered, and dressed in the morning. I go to bed at
whatever hour I want in the guest room and feel a great sense
of freedom because on those two nights I only have to take
care of me.

Despite the fact that Steven has MS, and each year he
needs help with more and more activities of daily living, our
relationship fortunately is still a partnership. The bonds and
the closeness that comes from sharing experiences, both
good and bad, in an open and honest way are there. There
is no question that I am his caregiver, but we still view ourselves as husband and wife. That being the case, I know I
have the right to let him know when the caregiving is just
getting too hard for me and we need to make some changes.
I don't do it often so when I do, Steven knows it is serious
and we have to find a way to relieve the pressure I am feeling

and the difficulties I am experiencing. And we do, not always easily, but we do.

The Guilt Factor

I never seem to find time for myself without wondering if she is okay.
—Rosie Miller, Phoenix, AZ

The fact that I tell Steven we need to make accommodations for me and he agrees doesn't mean it is a guilt-free experience. It is one thing to understand something intellectually. It's quite another to move beyond your emotional demons. If you feel guilty when you think about caring for yourself and taking a break, you are definitely not alone. Over the years I have heard many reasons given by family caregivers as to why they couldn't take a little time for themselves, why they couldn't spare time to protect their own health, why they couldn't ask someone else to take over part of their job. They include:

I'd worry all the time I was gone anyway, so why bother.
It wouldn't be right to do something just for me.
I know I should go to the doctor, but I am all doctored out.
I don't have the energy to exercise.
No one else could possibly care for John the way I do.
My mom would never let anyone else care for her.

If you feel guilty when you think about doing something that would be fun, or would give you an emotional or physical boost, think about the fact that even though you are providing care because you love and feel responsible for someone, much of the caregiving that you do is in fact a job, a job that other people get paid to perform. If caregiving was your

paid employment, if you were a doctor, nurse, physical therapist, short-order cook, or office administrator you would more
likely than not receive at least two weeks of vacation every
year, even though mandatory vacation is not required in the
United States. As a family caregiver you are in essence self-
employed. You aren't getting a salary and the job of caregiving
doesn't provide you with health insurance, but as your own
"boss" you can at least grant yourself some time off.

In Canada the law requires employers to provide employees ten days vacation with full pay. In the United
Kingdom mandatory vacation is twenty days, in France
and Sweden it's twenty-five, and in Austria and Finland it is
thirty days. That's actually good human resource policy. It
makes great business sense. People are more productive when
there is balance in their lives, when they take the time to "fill
up their tanks." But since this is America and as far as your
caregiving job goes, you are your own boss, it's up to you to
enforce a mandatory vacation rule for yourself, even if that
vacation is broken up into half-hour breaks every afternoon.
We all need a chance to rest, a change of scenery from time to
time, and we all need to enrich our lives by meeting new
people. Besides, have you ever considered that your loved
one might like a break from you and would appreciate seeing
and talking with others?

Barry Jacobs, PsyD, a clinical psychologist and family
therapist, is Director of Behavioral Sciences for the Crozer-
Keystone Family Medicine Residency Program in Springfield,
PA, and author of *The Emotional Survival Guide for
Caregivers*. According to Dr. Jacobs, caregiver guilt has several sources including an overpowering sense of obligation
that is sometimes heightened by admonitions from other family
members to keep up the good work. At times survivor guilt
comes into play. What did I do to cause this tragedy? What
didn't I do to prevent it? Because Mary can no longer play
golf, I'll give it up too.

I can relate to all of these reasons to feel guilty. My
mother-in-law, who died a few years ago, used to tell me how

wonderful I was and how much she loved me and appreciated so much what I did for Steven. I thought then, and still think now, about all the things I don't do that could possibly make life easier for her son. Whenever my manicurist tells me how special I am for staying with Steven, I feel as if I am being anointed with a sainthood I don't deserve. I've certainly been guilty of feeling guilty because I am glad that it isn't me who has MS, and I remember a period of time when I tried to live my life at Steven's pace so as not to leave him alone or leave him out of activities. In all of these instances the guilt didn't make me feel better. In fact it made me feel worse. That's because guilt is an insidious emotion that uses up a lot of energy to no purposeful end. It just makes a difficult situation even more difficult, and it certainly gets in the way of loving, honoring, and valuing yourself.

Respite

It isn't possible to talk about self-care for family caregivers without talking about respite. More than any other service, respite is what family caregivers want most. The primary purpose of respite care is to provide relief from the extraordinary and intensive demands of ongoing care to someone with special needs, thereby strengthening the family's ability to provide care. Respite care is planned and proactive. Respite means taking a break before extreme stress and crisis occurs.

A respite doesn't have to mean a week on the French Riviera, although that sounds pretty nice to me. It doesn't even have to be a weekend visiting friends, at least not at first. A respite can be as simple as lying on the couch with the lights dimmed listening to your favorite music, especially if you do it on a regular basis. It can be going to the movies or having a manicure every other week. You might even think of your three times a week exercise routine as a respite, if you enjoy it, rather than thinking of it as something you do because it is good for you.

I've come to think of respite as coming in three sizes, much the way things did in the house of the three bears that

Goldilocks visited. The week away is obviously comparable to a "papa bear" respite. A weekend visiting friends would fit nicely into "mama bear's" bowl, and all the little things that take an hour or less can be easily categorized as "baby bear" respites.

Truth be told, I've never taken a "papa bear" respite. The longest I've been away is four days and I had the built-in justification that it was for a business trip. But I have taken weekend respites, and each time I have reaped more benefits than I could have imagined. There was the weekend that Cindy and I went away and started to talk about our caregiving experiences. There was the weekend the following year when I went to the beach by myself and wrote the poem about the chair. I wrote another poem that weekend. There seems to be something about the salt air and the warmth of a summer breeze that nourishes my creative juices. The poem is called "Respite," and I've been told that it expresses the benefits that a weekend away can bring.

> *I rented a house at the beach this weekend.*
> *I went by myself and I took long walks*
> *I sat by an inlet of the bay and watched the reeds and*
> *intermittent trees, while they danced lightly in the breeze.*
> *I felt the sun's warmth on my face,*
> *and I willed it to seep deep into my soul.*
> *I went to the beach by myself this weekend.*
> *I was alone, but I was not lonely.*
> *I was with my self, and we were at peace—*
> *with each other.*

It's a wonderful feeling being with yourself. For me, it means living in the moment, breathing slowly and deeply, feeling a delightful sense of calm and warmth.

I can achieve some of these same feelings by indulging in my favorite "baby bear" respite, a bath by candlelight. Bubbles are a delightful addition, but they are optional. However, there is something about the glow of the candlelight that is essential to the experience because it somehow takes the edge off the responsibilities that lie just beyond the bathroom door. Warm water and soft lighting are sometimes enough for me, but at other times the addition of some calming music really helps take me away. It blocks out whatever household noises are invading my privacy and it involves yet another one of my senses in the experience. Touch, sight, sound, and sometimes taste and smell are added to my respite bath. A warm cup of tea gives me a glow on the inside just the way the warm bath water gives me a glow on the outside, and the scent of the tea, especially if it is a fruity blend is yet another way to further remove myself from the day-to-day demands. And every now and then I add the pièce de résistance, a piece of good quality chocolate. It does add a sort of decadent quality to the whole experience, and that is the point. I've come to the conclusion that if you are going to have a respite that only lasts fifteen or twenty minutes, it really should be decadent to have the proper effect.

I remember a time when I had been feeling fairly low and I mentioned it to a friend on the phone. A few days later a package arrived in the mail. When I opened it a huge smile spread across my face. Inside was a basket filled with everything I could possibly need for a delightful bathtub respite: bath oils, moisturizer, a big sponge, and lovely smelling soaps. It was such a thoughtful gift.

I know you may be thinking I am mad, but the point is it works for me. What you do on a respite break, regardless of its length, is up to you. It has to meet your needs, break your tensions, and renew your spirit. It needs to be the right medicine to cure, or at least ameliorate your current stress. It needs to be for you, precisely because you do so much for others and because you deserve it.

For my sixtieth birthday Steven gave me a gift certificate to a day spa, a big gift certificate, that allowed me to get a massage multiple times. I spread my visits to the spa out over the course of the next year. It truly was a gift that kept on giving. It was a gift that said, "Thank you for all you do for me. Now I want to give you something that, in its way, means I am taking care of you."

Next time you feel guilty for even thinking about taking a break, remember it is only partially for your benefit. Your loved one will reap a great deal of the benefit as well. Respites are guaranteed to take the edge off your tension, renew your energy, and give you a fresh dollop of patience with which to pick up your caregiving duties once again. Respite is the primary mechanism you have as a family caregiver to refill your tank and thereby keep on going. If you need proof, here it is.

> *Two family members volunteered to give us relief [from caring for my mom] for a week's family vacation. We had a wonderful time with our sons and came back refreshed.*
> —Ruthann S. McDonough, Carmel, IN

A number of studies have proven the value of respite to caregivers and their loved ones. A study looking at the benefits of respite for parents of children with emotional and behavioral disorders, published in 2000, shows that respite enhances the capacity to cope with stress, lessens the number of institutionalizations, and creates greater optimism about the caregiver's ability to continue to provide care.

Dr. Mary Mittleman of New York University has been studying spousal family caregivers of Alzheimer's patients for seventeen years and has found that respite and counseling lessens depression and helps caregivers avoid nursing home placement for their loved one for as much as a year and a half.

Practical Realities

Even if you want to take a weekend respite several times a year, or go to a weekly support group meeting, even if you truly believe self-care is a necessity, not a luxury, making it happen isn't always easy.

The survey of self-identified family caregivers revealed a disheartening fact. It found that even among family caregivers who believe strongly in the principle of caregiver self-care, there was often a disconnect between belief and action. Some of the survey questions were designed to gather data about the respondents' healthful activities both before and after becoming family caregivers. The answers to this series of questions were quite disturbing.

All of the respondents ate more nutritious meals, got more exercise, and went to see their doctor when they suspected a problem with their own health more often before becoming family caregivers than after. It wasn't because they didn't think it was important to continue these activities to the extent they did before. In fact, these caregivers said they thought it was extremely important that all family caregivers be told to preserve their own health. The survey didn't explore the reasons why the caregivers didn't or couldn't maintain their previous healthful behaviors, but I would surmise that it was because now that they had caregiving responsibilities they just felt they didn't have the time or energy to manage the logistics as easily as before. I certainly know that happens to me. Giving advice is a lot easier than following it yourself.

> *My body tells me I need a break, but I can't seem to find the resources to be able to do it.*
> —Jack Morris (Pseudonym), Orlando, FL

There probably isn't just one reason that caregivers spend little time caring for themselves. I know for myself that sometimes the thought of going to yet another doctor's appointment, even if it is to make sure that nothing is seriously wrong with me, is just too overwhelming. It means more time away from work. It means being in the milieu of medicine yet again. Sometimes I'm just too tired to get up and exercise. I'll shut off the alarm and hunker down under the covers for an extra thirty minutes of shut-eye, especially in the winter. It's easy to find an excuse not to do it. Life is more complicated than it used to be; time is more occupied with another's needs.

Wanting to do something and doing it are two totally differ-ent things. And the reasons you can't are, at times, out of your control.

Eleanor Cooney, a writer whose mother has Alzheimer's disease, angrily explained her point of view in an article in the October 2001 issue of *Harper's Magazine.*

> *Stability and predictability in daily routine are what the sages prescribe for people with Alzheimer's. They also have wise words for the caregivers: Take care of your-self. Give yourself a break. Be sure to set aside time do the things you enjoy. Get plenty of rest. Pamper your-self. Enlist the help of friends and relatives to assist with your "loved one." Take time out for yourself they chant. Time out for yourself? I'll let you in on a secret. There is no time out, not even when you are sound asleep, if the person is in fact a loved one and money is scarce.*

I suppose I am one of the sages that Eleanor is referring to. I certainly felt her anger jump off the page and punch me in the stomach the first time I read her words, and repeated readings haven't softened the blow. I understand her anger. I've had plenty of my own, but my anger wasn't focused on any particular message or human messenger, as hers is. I was angry at God.

I know many family caregivers, maybe some of you who are reading this book, share Eleanor's anger, and agree that I, and others who speak to and for family caregivers, are way off base. I respect your right to your anger, but I'd suggest it is misplaced. Your anger is better focused on the lack of support for caregiving families in our society. That is something we can change.

Eleanor referred to the scarcity of money being an issue for her, and rightly so. Research has shown that caregiving families tend to have lower household incomes than non-caregiving families and higher out of pocket expenses, as much as two and a half times higher by some accounts. You don't need to be an accountant to know that this type of cash flow situation isn't good for your financial health. According to the United States Census 2000, families in which one member has a disability have median incomes that are $15,360 less than non-caregiving families. It is not surprising, but is nevertheless shocking. In every single state, and Washington, DC, the poverty rate is higher among caregiving families than it is for the typical American family. Some caregivers leave the workforce. Others turn down promotions or decide to work part-time. All of this impacts income and benefits.

Most people's health insurance is part of their employment package if they are younger than age sixty-five, which is when we become eligible for Medicare, so the irony of being a family caregiver is that if you leave the workforce to take on the responsibility of giving care to someone whose own health is compromised, you may well be forced to compromise your ability to take care of your own. Add to that the fact that, as noted earlier, many products and services caregiving requires aren't covered by either private or government insurance. The inequities in the finances of caregiving families is an issue that has to be addressed if family caregivers are going to continue to be the primary providers of long-term care in our country.

In chapter three I wrote about how public policy impacts the daily lives of family caregivers and their loved one. The issue of caregiver finances is a perfect example. For some years now, members of Congress have introduced bills that would provide a tax credit for family caregivers providing the most intensive levels of care. Other pieces of proposed legislation would require social security credits for family caregivers who leave the work force, and other bills would have Medicare pay for adult daycare services. Does public policy affect the finances of caregiving families? Absolutely!

In addition to having limited finances, not having family or close friends nearby to help out can be a big factor in making it harder to "be for yourself." In some cases when money isn't the issue, finding people or services to hire is. Family caregivers usually have to compromise because our society isn't geared up to help us. More often than not we compromise ourselves. My point is that you can't always let that be the case because it can have dire effects not just for you, but for the very person you are trying to care for.

We need to harness Eleanor's words and anger, and the stories and frustration of many family caregivers and then we must use them, so that the idea of loving, honoring, and valuing ourselves is never seen as an expression created by blind idealists who don't have a clue what family caregiving is really about, but rather as a simple statement of the needs of family caregivers that can and must be met.

Things to Think, Permission to Do

Robert Bly wrote a poem that knocked me off my feet the first time I read it. It is a poem of great imagination. It is a poem of permission. It is a poem family caregivers should take to heart.

Things to Think

Think in ways you've never thought before.
If the phone rings, think of it as carrying a message,
Larger than anything you've ever heard,
Vaster than a hundred lines of Yeats.

Think that someone may bring a bear to your door,
Maybe wounded and deranged; or think that a moose
Has risen out of the lake, and he's carrying on his antlers
A child of your own whom you've never seen.

When someone knocks on the door, think that he's about
To give you something large: tell you you're forgiven,
Or that it's not necessary to work all the time or that it's
Been decided that if you lie down no one will die.

"If you lie down no one will die." Isn't that what we are afraid of in our heart of hearts? That if we are not there, something bad will happen and we'll never be able to forgive ourselves. We imagine the worst and create a prison that locks in our body, mind, and spirit. When we don't care for ourselves we are denying the possibility that good things are more likely to be the result than bad ones. When we don't care for ourselves we are doing a disservice to those we love as well as to ourselves. It is important to give yourself the gift of permission. Ultimately that is where loving, honoring, and valuing yourself has to begin. That's at the core of protecting your health.

Things to Think About, Things to Do

When was the last time you did something nice for yourself? When was the last time you took a real vacation? When was the last time you had a physical?

Have you ever said no to your loved one or a medical professional? If not, what would need to happen for you to consider it?

Do you now understand the connection between your good health, your energy level, and the quality of care you are able to provide? Since this is the first day of the rest of your life, what *realistic* new resolution can you put in place right away to begin to put that understanding into practice? Here are some ideas for things to do every day, every week, every month, and every year.

Every Day

Take a daily vitamin supplement: Being on the go often means we don't get our five-a-day fruits and vegetables. Taking a daily multivitamin supplement can fill in those gaps.

Brush and floss your teeth: When you are oh, so tired, it is understandable that you just may want to crawl into bed. Consider brushing and flossing your teeth right after dinner, when you aren't as wiped out.

Every Week

Exercise—even a little. It is one of the first things omitted from a busy caregiver's schedule. Physical caregiving can certainly provide some "incidental" exercise, but it is wise to try to get regular exercise as well. It's a great way to reduce stress and ward off depression. Could you allocate ten minutes three or four times a week to take a walk? Walking outside in good weather is nicest, but even power walking through your house and up and down some stairs will work. Start small. And don't beat yourself up if some weeks it doesn't happen. Just remember that it is really good for you and try to make it happen.

Find a caregiving buddy. Having another family caregiver to talk with can go a long way toward lessening your isolation. A buddy or a support group does just that—supports you, helps you think things through, helps you find new resources, and reminds you that others are experiencing the same or similar problems too.

Every Month

Get away from your caregiving to have some fun at least once a month, but ideally more than that. Whether it is dinner with friends, a manicure, or a massage, doing something for you will make you feel so much better.

Add some spirituality to your life. Whether it is through reading poetry or going to church, we all need to renew our soul and our connection to something larger than ourselves. Try to do this as often as you can.

Every Year

Get a flu shot. The Centers for Disease Control and Prevention (CDC) puts family caregivers in the second-highest-risk group in terms of priority status for obtaining a flu shot. Our chronically ill loved ones are in the first group. Since we are out and about mingling with others, we could bring the flu home and infect our loved ones; and because they depend on us for care, keeping us flu-free is considered really important as well. Now more than ever, with concerns about a flu pandemic, getting your flu shot is one of the most important things you can do to protect your health and your loved one's.

Have an annual physical: The last place you want to spend time is another doctor's office, but taking the time for a checkup once a year could save you countless hours in doctors' offices later. Small problems that go undetected and untreated can turn into big problems that threaten your life. For women, an annual Pap smear and, "if you are of a certain age," a mammogram is absolutely critical. Make it a point to tell your doctor that you are a family caregiver and how that is affecting you—your mood, sleeping and eating patterns, your back, and so on.

Have a real respite: Going to a movie is great, but to get a real respite that renews your spirit and your soul it is important to have a change of venue. A week or two away would be fantastic, but is totally unrealistic for most of us. Even a weekend may be hard to pull off, but the effort it takes to make it happen can pay huge dividends. Another option is to check into a local hotel for one night. You may still be in the same city, but you'll feel miles away and that is what counts. If you can't afford a hotel, perhaps a friend will let you spend the night in her spare room. We all need a break from our loved ones once in a while—and they need a break from us as well.

It's not easy to take care of yourself when you are a family caregiver, but it is so important to try. Don't let misplaced guilt sideline you. You work so hard and do so much and you are doing the very best you can. Your effort and your sacrifices need to be acknowledged. Because you need to be there for someone else, the importance of taking care of *you* becomes doubly important. Some days, some weeks, some months, you'll let self-care activities slide. We all do. It's only natural. The challenge we all face is not letting the down times outnumber the times we are actively doing something that is healthful and helpful. Not easy, but we do need to try. (If it makes you feel any better I am sitting at my desk working on this book, when I had actually planned to be doing some exercise. It's Sunday and a beautiful spring day. I tell myself, later I will go for a walk.)

~~ CHAPTER 6 ~~

Help Is Not a Dirty Word

Find help as soon as you can. If you refuse help nicely in the beginning, people will never ask you again.
— Barb Stutzka, West Concord, MN

Why is it so hard to ask for help? What's a good response to the statement, "Call me if you need me"? How is it that despite the fact that we are drowning in responsibility or are really confused about what our next step should be, we often respond with "no thanks" when help is offered? Where do we find help if we decide we need it, and what can we do about those siblings of ours who refuse to help out with Mom and Dad?

Asking for and accepting help is a complex issue. Obviously, we first need to recognize that having some help can make a real difference to our loved one's wellbeing and ours as well. Then we need to figure out what we actually need help with and what kind of help we are willing to accept. There are also practical issues to consider regarding paid help versus friendly help. If this just sounds like more work, another list of things to do, know that it doesn't have to be an overwhelming task, but rather just a way to organize thoughts and information you already have.

Just as with respite, which is designed to give you a relaxing break from your responsibilities, help can restore your

123

equilibrium by removing some responsibility from your shoulders, and lessening your stress. Help will also enable you to be a more peaceful and effective caregiver. The science shows it will certainly make you a healthier person. It is precisely because you do care that getting help when you need it is important.

Not all family caregivers need help. If your husband is relatively independent despite his disability, or your dad just needs a daily reminder to take his medications, then your caregiving responsibilities may well be very manageable and not an issue of concern at this time. But for those who need to help loved ones with personal care on a daily basis, or are part of the sandwich generation caring for elders as well as kids, or are just feeling generally overwhelmed by caregiving issues, having help can make a big difference.

The Benefits of Having Help

- It can lessen your sense of isolation knowing that other people have an idea of what you are dealing with and are willing to be there for you when needed.
- It can move the dial on your "worry meter" down to a safe level.
- It can encourage your loved one to be more independent.
- It can give you more confidence in your ability to manage your caregiving responsibilities.
- It can increase your ability to think creatively and expand the options you now have available to you.

To my way of thinking, those are pretty good benefits indeed.

If you can think of some other ones, write them down on a piece of paper, or print them off of your computer, along with the ones that I have listed. Stick them on your refrigerator door or some other place where you will see them often. Since asking for help is often such a hard thing to do, we need all the encouragement we can get to do it.

Barriers to Seeking and Accepting Help

The hardest part is fear, fear of refusal, fear of being misunderstood, or fear that I'll be considered whiny.

　　　　　　　—E. Dee Manies, Overland Park, KS

Why is it so darn hard? What prevents us from reaching out or letting others in? I think it has a lot to do with pride because, in addition to helping us recognize our accomplishments and encouraging us to persevere, pride can impede relationships and close us off from others. Pride swells our hearts when our children bring home a report card filled with As, and pride in ourselves is part of the reward for learning a new computer program or losing those five pounds that we gained last Christmas. But pride can get in the way when it is the cause of our refusing to apologize to a friend for a hurtful act, or when it won't let us admit we made a bad decision. In the context of caregiving, pride can prolong the time we struggle before we seek assistance, and it can get in the way of accepting help even when it is sincerely offered and very concrete. For men this can be a particular problem since many men think they are always supposed to be strong and silent in the face of adversity.

The hardest part about asking for help was shedding the cultural conditioning that men are tough, that men don't cry, that real men don't eat quiche and they should be able to handle whatever life throws their way.

　　　　　　　—Ron Perry, Wayne, PA

As Americans we are brought up to be fiercely independent and for many of us, very private about our personal lives too. Asking for help forces us to admit we can't do everything ourselves and necessitates that we peel away some of the layers that protect our private lives from public view.

These are not easy things to do. They take time, and doing them often embarrasses us. But once we work through our pride, or at least the portion of it that impacts our willingness to ask for and receive assistance, our lives and those of our loved ones can be more enjoyable, less scary, and a great deal safer.

It's good to remember that in many circumstances it isn't only our pride that must be dealt with. Your husband may be adamant about not wanting someone else to touch his genitals. Your siblings may repeatedly dissuade you from letting others know the true circumstances of your mom's dementia. Pride is about self-image, and taking steps that will potentially alter your self-image or the image you, your loved one, and your family project to the world is a big deal. So much of caregiving occurs behind the closed doors of bedrooms and bathrooms. No wonder we are hesitant to ask for help.

What we need to understand is that there are all sorts of ways that other people can help without seeing the most private details of our caregiving. In other cases it is those personal details that we need help with the most. Somewhere along the line we have to strike a balance between independence and practicality.

Caregiving Is Work

As family caregivers we are adding work to our already busy lives, and even though most of us very willingly and lovingly take on this added responsibility, it is important to remember that it is just that, more responsibility and more work. So what happens to all of the other work currently on your plate? Cooking and cleaning and shopping, being a carpool mom for the kids, walking the dog, holding down a job, paying the bills, none of these are going away.

If you can find even one person or one service that can reduce your regular workload by either taking over all or part of one of your regular chores, you'll have more time for your caregiving, and less stress bearing down on you. If you can find a person or service that can help with your specific caregiving responsibilities, you'll be in a better position to meet your non-caregiving responsibilities. Finding help is often difficult for emotional, financial, and geographic reasons, but it can make a big difference in your ability to be an effective caregiver; it can make a big difference in your loved one's wellbeing; and it can make a difference in your own wellbeing and that of other family members as well. It's worth the effort.

Defining the Help You Need

When people offer to help, be ready to give them a date and time when they are needed.
— Dick Stone, Oklahoma City, OK

Getting help requires creativity and perseverance. You first need to define what you need help with, which tasks or chores would be the easiest to get others to help with, which you really want to do yourself, and which if any you can afford to pay others to do. And then there is the actual reaching out and opening up. You don't need to do it all at once. In fact I wouldn't recommend it. Take it a step at a time so you can get comfortable with the whole idea.

If you are willing to plunge in, defining the help you need could actually be one of the first things you get help with. What about asking a friend to help you think through your list of responsibilities and put some ideas on paper, or if he or she knows you fairly well, perhaps he or she will even begin a list for you? At times that little jumpstart is what it takes, especially if you are like the 38 percent of responding caregivers in a 1997 survey by the National Alliance for Caregiving and AARP who said they didn't know what kind of help would benefit them.

Over the years, I've developed a process to define the help I need. It does require, at least the first few times you do it, making lists; I want to say that upfront. But it really isn't an onerous task and I find it useful to this day. In fact, I find when I do make the effort to put things down on paper, rather than just think about them in my head, I have the opportunity to keep the list as a living document that I can add to when I have new thoughts. Inevitably when I go through this process I gain insights that eventually move me to take action, which really is the whole point of making the list in the first place.

A Recipe for Defining and Getting Help

Step 1

Recognize that caregiving, like all jobs, is made up of many individual tasks, not all of which are of the same importance. Some tasks take a few minutes while others may take many hours. Some tasks are easy; others require skill and fortitude. The challenge is to know the difference.

Step 2

Recognize that asking for help is a sign of strength and not of weakness. It means you truly have a grasp on your situation and have come up with a proactive problem-solving technique to try to make things easier or better.

Step 3

Start a list of all your caregiving-related tasks for any given week (or at least those you are most concerned about), such as filing insurance forms; arranging your schedule to meet work obligations and still be able to take your son to counseling three times a week; getting nutritious meals on the table most nights; and lifting, bathing, dressing, and undressing your husband. When you see the types of tasks that are on your list you'll realize there is a good reason why you are so tired and don't have time for yourself. If this is proving difficult for you perhaps the following chart, which lists some specific needs and also some corresponding ways that friends, family, or volunteers could meet them, might help.

A Caregiver's List of Needs	*How Friends or Family Can Help*
A ride to doctor appointments every other Monday	"Chauffeur Service" at a preassigned date and time
Getting dinner on the table	A meal prepared and delivered on Tuesdays and Thursdays for the next three months
Dealing with the insurance company	Forms filled out monthly as well as several hours of my time each month to advocate on your behalf
Someone to care about me	A weekly phone call, a shoulder to cry on
Keeping the house clean	A maid brigade every other week, until school starts
Keeping food in the house	Doing the grocery shopping every week for the next two months
Emergency assistance	My commitment to come when you call
Some quiet time alone	Taking Paul out for a ride every other Saturday
Help with household maintenance	A promise to mow your lawn all summer and the availability of my tools and time if we can schedule it in advance

Con't. on page 130

A Caregiver's List of Needs	How Friends or Family Can Help
More time	Running weekly errands for you, going to the drugstore, the cleaners, and taking Betty to Sunday school
More money	I can't write you a check but I can go to the discount store and buy you things in bulk
A homecare aide	My commitment to coordinate a volunteer team from the church to help out with specific caregiving tasks

Step 4

I am a big believer in organizing ideas into categories. It helps me see the big picture and understand how individual activities fit into the puzzle that comprises the caregiving aspects of my life. Categories may include personal-care tasks for your loved one, transportation, and household chores. You may think that all your tasks fit neatly into only a few categories, or you may be more comfortable with being more specific and thereby have many more categories into which your individual tasks fall. There's no right or wrong method. It's all a matter of personal preference.

Step 5

What do you worry about most as a family caregiver? Who will help Mom if she falls and no one is around? Where will we get the money to pay for John's medications? Who will care for Mary if I get sick? Where can I find affordable daycare? If you are like me, your worries fit into one of the same categories as your tasks. I think it's important to be able to name your worries. Speaking them out loud or seeing them circled on a piece of paper somehow transforms them from abject fears to problems to be solved. That's a more comfortable place for me. It doesn't make my big worries disappear, but at least it lets me approach them in a somewhat rational way. It lets me see them in a different light, and gives me hope that I can find a way to deal with them, rather than paralyzing me into doing nothing until they turn into crises and I am forced to do something.

Step 6

Whenever I go through this process of defining my needs, which is usually when I sense things are beginning to unravel, I feel so much better. It gives me a sense of satisfaction and even relief, as if I've seen a storm coming and I've managed to get home just before the downpour begins. It let's me say that if I try I just may be able to keep my head above water yet again. It's a calming feeling, one that lets me look at my list of tasks and worries with a less emotional eye and admit which tasks I actually like doing; which I hate or feel incompetent to deal with well; which I really think I have to do myself, at least for the time being; and which are simply ho-hum things that have to be done, but don't carry any particular emotional impact one way or the other. It helps me think about what tasks I should seek assistance with, which, if any, I can afford to pay someone else to do, or which I might ask a friend or family member, neighbor, or even a volunteer team from the synagogue to help me out with.

Perhaps helping your mom with her shower falls into the "I have to do it myself" category, whereas taking her to a regular doctor's appointment is something you can envision someone else doing. Do you enjoy cooking or the time you spend helping your daughter exercise her legs? What can't you stand dealing with or feel insecure about?

Is going to the supermarket or managing your brother's medications on your list of things that need to get done but that are no big deal to you? As you are thinking about this, please make sure that not everything falls under the "I have to do it myself" category. The idea here is to get a handle on how you can lessen your load, not keep it the same.

Here's my current list. It is different from the one that appeared in the first edition of this book. At that time I was taking care of all of Steven's personal-care needs myself. I wasn't feeling overly burdened by them. Then the kind of help I focused on was assistance with housecleaning and maintenance issues, such as mowing the lawn and keeping the gutters clear. Today I still need help with those items, and unfortunately Steven needs significantly more personal-care help as well.

After I prepared my earlier list and shared it with Steven, we came to the conclusion that we really needed to meet with a financial planner. Now we have one and believe we are making much sounder decisions because of it. A lot changes in five years and so some of the items on my current list didn't appear on the earlier one. Steven is talking about retirement now and we renovated the house to make it fully accessible and plan to say in it as long as we possibly can. Both of these things have major implications in the short and long term. Life goes on. Things change and with them our list of tasks, our attitudes toward them, and our worries and fears.

We are much more fortunate than many caregiving families. Now we can afford to purchase some of the help we need, but it definitely involves making some serious choices. I know Steven's need for personal-care services is only going to increase. Down the line we will have to review the decisions we've made recently and reassess our priorities.

Suzanne's List of Major Tasks, Attitudes, and Worries		
Tasks	**Attitudes** *Like (L); Dislike/No Time (DL/ NT); Must Do Myself (MDM); Ho Hum (HH)*	**Worries**
Steven's Personal Care: Category A		
1. Transfers: morning, evening, in the bathroom 2. Showering 3. Dressing 4. Toileting 5. Catheterizing 6. Eating	DL/MDM: We have help now two nights a week and that is making a big difference but it doesn't solve our emergency situations.	How do I make things as tolerable for Steven as possible when I'm traveling? How will we handle all of the personal-care items when Steven can't participate at all in his own care? The biggest worry for me, and the one I can't do anything about is: will the MS stay confined to general bodily movement or will it attack his eyes? Will it affect him cognitively? Is our emergency network of neighbors secure and large enough so that we don't wear out our welcome if Steven should need help on a regular basis for a while, as he did when he had bladder surgery?
7. Medication Management	HH	

Con't. on page 134

Household Chores: Category B		
1. Cooking	L	
2. Food Shopping	L	
3. Laundry	HH	
4. Housework 5. Gardening/Lawn Maintenance 6. House Maintenance	DL/NT	We are lucky. A housekeeper comes once a week. The worry is: will it become too expensive for us to stay in the house? We've made the decision we want to stay here and "age in place."
Finances: Category C		
1. Income in Retirement	We have a financial planner now whom we trust. He's doing what he can to help us have the best nest egg we can.	Will we be able to afford even more home care when Steven needs it? It's very expensive and now we are both still working.
2. File Insurance Claims	DL: Right now we only have one to file so it isn't a big deal.	Will filing insurance claims become a big part of our life in the future? I have "form phobia."
3. Banking	HH: We bank online now. It saves lots of time and makes it easier to stay on top of bills.	

Step 7

If you are comfortable doing it, I'd suggest sharing these thoughts with a close family member, a good friend, another caregiver, or perhaps your clergyman or the employee-assistance counselor at work. I'd advise discussing them with your care recipient if that is possible. The intent here isn't necessarily to get actual physical help or professional advice, but to let you have the benefit of hearing other people's ideas and insights. Two brains focused on solving a problem is usually more effective than one!

Step 8

As the folks at Nike say, "Just Do It!" Take a deep breath and actually ask someone to help with one of the tasks on your list, or ask for guidance in resolving your most persistent worry. I'd suggest starting with something small, especially if you are looking for hands-on assistance or something that requires someone doing you a favor. It might take a few times before you begin to get comfortable with the idea. With practice, it really does get easier. Just one more bit of advice on this score, I promise. Don't forget to be open to those offering to help. With your list of tasks in hand and your sense of your priorities and concerns, you'll be better able to take advantage of opportunity when it knocks. You'll have a ready response when someone says, "Call me if you need me." You'll be able to say, "I would really like to find a pharmacy that delivers, but I just haven't had the time to do the research, would you be willing to do it for me?"

Help Can Come in Many Forms

The kind of help we need most these days falls into three categories: assistance with household maintenance, personal care for Steven, and transportation assistance so he can continue to go to work a couple of days a week. I enjoy cooking, and can certainly handle the laundry and other basic household chores, but I am not handy when it comes to fix-it things. I don't really enjoy gardening, and quite frankly I don't have the time given my other priorities. We are very fortunate that we can have someone mow the lawn, clean the house, and, most recently, help Steven with personal tasks twice a week. Steven and I have agreed that as long as we can continue to pay for those services we will.

But there is some help that no amount of money can buy. It's the help I need when Steven falls during a transfer, especially when it's a transfer from toilet to wheelchair and he ends up on the cold tile floor of the bathroom. It's real-time emergency help I need then, and it necessitates that I rely on others. That's when I give Warren or Tony a call.

Warren is one of our neighbors. He lives directly across the street. He's tall, well over six feet, solid, and in his early thirties. Somehow, miraculously it seems to me, Warren is usually available when I need his help. I've come to think of Warren as my knight in shining armor who comes over at a moment's notice and with a few deft strokes manages to pick Steven up and right him in his wheelchair. It's such a comfort knowing that Warren lives across the street and is so willing to literally lend a hand.

It took a lot for us to get over the pride and the embarrassment of having to ask for help in such personal circumstances, and we didn't do it easily. I recall one time when Steven fell and we were still trying to deal with such situations on our own. I used a sheet to drag him from the bathroom, across the wooden floor and down the hall, past the guest room and his office, and then onto the carpeting in the master bedroom.

There was no place at all in the bathroom that he could hold on to, and from which I could try to bend his legs and position them in such a way that working together we could maneuver him into a standing position. At least in our bedroom there was the fairly low platform bed frame with decorative cutouts that work well as hand holds. First I had to get Steven's body in a straight line so I could get the sheet under him sufficiently enough to carry him along as I dragged it, huffing and puffing, toward the bedroom. It required strength I really didn't have.

Once in the bedroom we struggled and struggled to control the spasticity in his legs, bend his knees, and raise enough of his upper body to the bed to allow me to lift his lower body and legs on the bed, and then transfer him back into the wheelchair as we did each morning. The whole process took about forty-five exhausting minutes to go a distance of just twenty-three feet. Steven's skin was rubbed raw and my back was sore. That was it. We weren't going to try that ever again. Reality was pushing pride aside. We agreed we needed to reach out to neighbors, and so that's what we started to do.

I'm actually very lucky. If Warren isn't home, I know I can always turn to Tony who lives next door. Tony isn't quite as tall as Warren, and he's definitely older, but he too is quite strong, and most importantly, always so willing to help at a moment's notice.

Steven had bladder surgery some years ago. In the scheme of things it was a relatively minor operation, but given his disability it totally destroyed whatever strength he had to help himself, especially because there was now a row of stitches across his abdomen. Bending from the waist was particularly painful and there was no way we could get him in and out of bed each morning and night using our usual transfer technique. Insurance wasn't willing to pay for homecare assistance so we had to find help on our own.

The first night Steven was home from the hospital I asked Tony if he would be willing to come over and help me get Steven into bed. "Of course I'll come. What time?" he said. He came that night at 10:15 and the next morning at 6:30, and he continued to come morning and night for the next five days, until we felt comfortable doing the transfer on our own, but he made me promise I wouldn't hesitate to call if we needed his help again. He was embarrassed when I kept telling him how grateful I was. "Don't think about it. That's what neighbors are for. I'm glad to help, really," he said. And I knew he meant it.

I recall one Sunday afternoon when Steven had slipped out of his wheelchair during a transfer (we seemed to go through a period of several months before we had come to terms with the fact that the stair glide we had installed to get Steven from house to garage and back again was no longer working for us, and thus we were experiencing the consequences) and neither Warren nor Tony was at home. Unfortunately, neither was Kathy or Phil, or Debra who I've also called on from time to time. It seemed we were the only ones around on that lovely sunny Sunday. Bereft of neighbors, or at least those I felt comfortable enough asking at the time, I called the fire department. If people ask them to get cats out of trees, I surmised, they can surely help lift a man off of the floor. Sure enough, three members of the rescue squad showed up within fifteen minutes. "Any time ma'am," they said with a smile.

I've become very good at asking for help, in putting necessity first and pride last. I've learned that caregiving is more than a one-person job and that I need to know when something is beyond my capabilities. I've learned how absolutely critical it is to make a conscious effort to create a network of support, to have people I can call on in an emergency. I've also learned it doesn't just happen. It requires an effort and a breaking down of barriers. I had to let people into my life and Steven's, to tell our story, to let them see my vulnerability as well as my strength. It's the price family caregivers have to pay, but the rewards are well worth it.

We've gotten to know a few more people in the neighborhood lately. Two of them work near Steven and now that he now longer drives they've agreed to each drive him to work one day a week in our accessible minivan. Arthur lives a few doors away, and he literally works right across the street from Steven. He's the first person I asked if he'd be willing to be Steven's driver. We met Dennis at a party the weekend before I put a note out on our neighborhood listserv to find a second driver. Talk about serendipity. He responded to my listing, said he passed Steven's building everyday and would be happy to drive one day a week. Dennis has a next-door neighbor who we know by sight. I stop and pet his dog when he walks by and we have chatted briefly. He seems really nice, the kind of guy who would be willing to be part of our emergency team. I know he wants to see our renovation, and Steven and I love to show the house off, so I plan on inviting him and his wife over for a tour, and shortly after that I'll ask him.

When yours is a caregiving family, you can't have too many people on your list of emergency helpers.

Thoughts on Where to Look for Help

The person who says, "I have two hours on Friday afternoon or Saturday morning . . . could I pick up your children and take them to the park?" or "I would love to come on Thursday and bring dinner, if you would like." . . . These folks are angels in disguise.
— K. Metzguer, Hillsborough, NC

The number of things family caregivers need help with is seemingly endless. There is no one solution that is right for everyone. Where you live may well be a factor, as may your income (too high for government programs, too low to allow you to pay for services). Nevertheless, here are some possible directions.

Perhaps there are county services such as Meals on Wheels that can bring nourishing food to your dad every day, so that you don't have to drive over to him as often. Perhaps you can rearrange your work schedule to have a half-day off every Friday afternoon during which to deal with your sister's appointments and insurance paperwork.

Is there a parish nurse service available in your area? Can you afford to hire a homecare aide for several hours a week to give your partner a bed bath? Will your best friend's teenage son mow your lawn in the summer and shovel the snow from your driveway in the winter? If you live in Los Angeles and your parents live in Omaha can you find a geriatric-care manager there to assess your parents' situation and provide you with weekly reports? Might a nursing student be willing to watch your disabled child once a week so you can more easily run errands?

Will your brother agree to help finance your mom's care, if you agree to be the primary caregiver? Will your neighbors agree to pitch in and bring over meals four times a week so you don't have to think about what's for dinner?

Technology is playing an ever-expanding role in finding ways to assist family caregivers and their loved ones. Equipment for monitoring Mom's daily activities and equipment to monitor your spouse's vital signs are available, and new ideas for equipment to help with toileting and bathing functions are appearing. I saw a video a few years ago about an experimental robotic nurse/companion—an R2D2 for the over-eighty set. The prototype looked great and perhaps we'll see the "nursebot" in actual use in the not too distant future.

I asked some longstanding family caregivers for their advice on where to find help. Here's what they said.

> *Begin by finding out what is available from the health insurance company, Medicare, or Medicaid. Then check with state programs, community services, and church programs in your community. . . . With planning and organization you can work toward having the help you need.*
>
> —Linda Reid, Oneonta, AL

> *I've asked at the local privately owned drug store, asked neighbors, asked nurses at my husband's dialysis clinic.*
>
> —Paulette Miley, Chesnee, SC

> *When I saw what was coming, I immediately increased our world and put us in a position to meet more people. Mainly church groups, etc.*
>
> —J. Tjugum, Hartland, WI

In Appendix A I listed a variety of organizations including their national phone numbers and Web site addresses, but it is important to remember that ultimately the resources you are most likely to need are local. The purpose of giving you these national contacts is so that you will have a starting point from which to begin your search.

Also consider volunteer networks. There are several models that have a proven track record. Sheila Warnock and the late Cappy Capossela were so profoundly affected by their experience as part of a group of ten other women who came together to care for a friend dying of cancer that they documented their experience as well as the systems and forms they used in a book titled *Share the Care*. As word spread other people wanted to develop volunteer caregiving families. Since the book was published more than 97,000 people have participated in Share the Care groups. To learn more about the book and the organization it spawned go to: www.sharethecare.org

There are Web-based programs that have been developed based on the same premise; no one person should bear the entire load. The Web site www.lotsahelpinghands.com relies on a friend or family member to coordinate a volunteer-helper team. This person posts listings of what the family needs on any given day: meals, a ride to the doctor, some handyman services, or help with doing nighttime transfers. The coordinator finds someone from the list of people who have agreed to participate, who can do what is needed at the time needed, schedules it and sends out reminders, too. This Web-based model is efficient and easy to use. Its scheduling function lets everyone know who's on tap for what and when. It also provides a speedy way to find out who is available in an emergency or who is available to replace someone who just can't help out on Tuesday as they had said they would.

A Cautionary Note

I wish I could say that making lists and knowing people and places to reach out to guarantees that you will definitely get help, but unfortunately that isn't the case. What it does do is put you in a much better position to get assistance than you would have been in if you hadn't gone through the process. But it is important to be realistic. There will definitely be disappointments.

> *People are very kind, but they will not show up. They are busy; they are sick, they are over committed. Probably they are scared to see him being so disabled.*
> —L. Brown, Richmond, CA

*The hardest part is not getting it [help] after finally
working up the nerve to ask for it.*
                    —Susan Kiser Scarff, Phoenix, AZ

All in the Family

If you have family members who help you out with your
caregiving responsibilities, you are very fortunate. Many people
don't. Helping each other can bring close families even closer.
It can be a catalyst that helps build strong bonds that continue even after the caregiving experience is over. In families
where there traditionally have been tensions it can help ease
them, but unfortunately the opposite is definitely true as well.

Steven and I are lucky in that regard; our daughter,
Darryn, and son-in-law Steve (note the use of the nickname,
that's how we distinguish between the two) live just ten minutes away. Darryn is often available to help out if I have a
dinner meeting downtown or some other engagement that
throws off my set schedule. She'll stop by on her way home
from work and get Steven his dinner, which I have ready in
the refrigerator. She only needs to heat it up in the micro-
wave, set the table, and get him a glass of juice. If she brings
Kaylyn with her, Steven has the pleasure of seeing his daughter
and granddaughter, and I have the piece of mind that comes
from knowing things are under control.

Darryn often asks me to help her out as well and I like
that. It makes ours a symbiotic relationship. We each help
each other. Sometimes she'll ask me to stop by her house at
lunchtime and let the dog in if it looks like it will rain, and
sometimes she asks me to babysit, or attend a function at
Kaylyn's school, which I love to do.

If your family doesn't help out, though, realize you are
not alone. In most families one of the "kids" is providing the
bulk of care for Mom or Dad. This can range from being the
prime decision-maker or the major hands-on caregiver. A great
way for families to stay in touch with each other and for the
primary caregiver to give others a day-by-day update, thereby
building a real picture of what actually is happening, is to
create a family Web site. The Web site www.carepages.com is

one of a number of online mechanisms for building community when a family member is ill. It permits back-and-forth communications among the participants, the opportunity to post pictures or documents, and it saves the family caregiver the effort of updating everyone individually.

Spousal caregivers and parents whose children have special needs are often going it alone, too. In some situations spousal caregivers don't want to let their children know how difficult things are. I often hear, "They have their own families to worry about. I couldn't possibly ask them for help. I don't want to burden them with my problems." Parents of children with special needs get more help from other family members than other types of caregivers, but it often peters out as the child gets older and is often non-existent when the child becomes an adult.

The reasons for this are as complicated as the family dynamics involved. Some families are close and have always reached out to each other. Others are barely on speaking terms. Siblings have rivalries. Adult children are estranged. Parents are divorced. And there are those of us who think we shouldn't have to ask family. Family members ought to recognize we need help and offer.

> *My brothers and sister helped out when they could, but even though I was feeling totally desperate, I felt that I should not be asking for help and did not share how bad things had gotten.*
> —Melissa McKerrow, Rockville, MD

A Family Meeting

Getting family members to help you is not an impossible task. However, it isn't fair to think that everyone can read your mind, especially if they live far away and don't see what actually is involved. That's why professionals often say the most important thing to do is have a family meeting, and to have the first one as early in the caregiving process as possible. This will allow everyone to understand the situation and what is likely to happen in the future.

Having the meeting in person is ideal, because you can

see each other's facial expressions and body language. Making an effort to get to the meeting place shows a commitment at least to take a real look at the issues, and it can be an opportunity for family members who haven't been together in a while to reunite around a common concern. However, if an in-person meeting is impossible consider telephone conferencing, or, if everyone is online, e-mail, instant messaging, or a private chat room. If done early, it can preclude one person unwittingly having to carry the bulk of the caregiving alone. If you are already that bulk-carrying caregiver, the meeting is a mechanism to help you lighten your load.

You'll need to decide whether or not the care recipient should be present. That will depend on their state of mind and whether or not he or she is resistant to having help. The advantage to having everyone at the meeting is that you are all involved and can have your say. The meeting is not supposed to lead to a family conspiracy against the person who needs care. Its goal is exactly the opposite, to bring you all closer together and come up with a sound plan for helping you and managing the care of your loved one. If having a family meeting sounds like an idea you'd like to try, here are some tips to keep in mind.

- Plan ahead; give yourself time to prepare. Suggest several alternate dates.
- It's a good idea to have a facilitator at the meeting, especially if you think the meeting is likely to be divisive. A trusted member of the clergy, a social worker, geriatric care manager, or nurse who is familiar with your care recipient's condition are all good choices. That person can keep the conversation on track, take notes, referee if voices are raised, provide an impartial point of view, and share information about your loved one's illness, the realities of insurance coverage, and long-term care financing. They can also touch on the mounting emotional stress of caregiving that everyone will have to deal with as time goes by.

- At the meeting it is perfectly okay to have a written list outlining key points you want to make. It won't ruin your credibility. On the contrary, it will show that you've thought this through carefully.
- When describing your situation, be as specific as possible. Try drawing a verbal picture of a typical day. Use imagery and statistics to make your points memorable.
- Get feedback. If people aren't offering any, the facilitator's job is to stir conversation. If there is no facilitator involved, then you'll have to take the lead by saying, "I'd like to know what you're thinking or feeling." Don't be surprised if some people are in denial, and others are nervous or defensive. People need time to absorb all you've said, but they should be reminded that if something happened to you, someone else would have to step in. Better to preclude that from happening by working out a shared caring plan now.
- It's good to add a little levity to the situation. Humorous anecdotes and jokes can break the tension and preserve everyone's dignity. The facilitator can both initiate this and draw the group back to the discussion at hand.
- At the end of the meeting it is important to have closure. What has been decided? Will there be another meeting? If so, who is in charge of arranging it? As the organizer of the first meeting you should send out a memo listing the key points of the discussion and next steps, or you might ask the facilitator to do it. Agree to stay in touch by whatever means are most practical. You've started a dialogue. It is important to keep it going.
- End with a pizza or some other prepared meal. Sitting around the table together is a good reminder that this was a family meeting, not a business one. If time and energy allow, perhaps the help could begin that very day with Nancy gathering the insurance policies to review, and Dave raking the leaves from the lawn.

An Asking-for-Help Success Story

Sue Tissian is a caregiver for her husband, Sam, who had a stroke a few years ago. She hadn't told anyone how she felt about her changed life until she decided to respond to an NFCA request for family caregivers to share their stories and a list of needs and wishes that would make their caregiving situation better.

Something inside her told Sue it was time to take a look at her concerns. She sat down and wrote her story—just five short paragraphs and a needs-and-wishes list of four items. It wasn't easy to do, she told us. It brought a lot of emotions to the surface and it made her admit how difficult it was to be a family caregiver. Once it was done, however, she felt better, and so decided to show it to her daughter Marlene.

> *I am a 73 year old healthy woman, caring for my 74 year old spouse. Though I have some physical problems of my own, they take a back seat to the needs of my husband, Sam. His stroke left him with a right side weakness which [sic] requires him to use a walker and severe aphasia and apraxia. [Aphasia is the loss or impairment of the power to use words. Apraxia is the inability to execute complex coordinated movements]. Though he uses Metro Access for his weekly speech therapy sessions, I drive him to wherever his needs take us. I now manage all household, financial, physical, and communication needs for both of us.*
>
> *I feel overwhelmed most of the time and accomplish very little except meeting our immediate needs. He does not require constant care. He is capable of caring for himself almost completely so I can leave him for long periods, but I feel guilty whenever I do.*
> *Another difficult adjustment for me is the autonomous decision-making. This is no longer a shared responsibility; it has become a very heavy burden.*

We would like to move to more accessible living quarters because I can no longer maintain the grounds and repairs on this aging house, but the thought of getting rid of 48 years of accumulated junk puts me in a state of immobility.

After over 50 years of marriage, I find that I am not the strong burden carrier I always thought I was. I miss our conversations, our spontaneous activities and our independence.

If I had a dream list, it would include some of the following:

1. The sale of our house.
2. Finding and moving to a new home.
3. Traveling again, whenever the desire arose.
4. Another regular exercise program that he would enjoy.

As soon as Marlene read her mom's story, she and her husband Barry leapt into action. They hired a realtor and within six weeks, Sue's home had been sold and a new home in a well-run retirement community had been found. Marlene and Barry took care of all the details. Sue's job was to make the final decisions and sign the papers.

I had no idea about the depth of mom's anguish or that the reason she hadn't sold the house was because she perceived it to be an enormous task to move. Whenever we were together she was in good spirits. She seemed to be coping with whatever things life threw at her. I wish I would have known just how important it was for her to move.

Selling the house was not a difficult task for us to take care of. I'm just glad she finally shared her story with us.

Afterword

It's been more than thirty years since Steven was diagnosed with multiple sclerosis, and sixteen years since Cindy and I began to talk about finding a way to help family caregivers. I never could have imagined at either of those times how each event would affect my life and those of so many other people.

I am grateful for how I have grown as a person because of both of these events, and I am humbled by the achievements of NFCA and the knowledge that this organization Cindy and I began has become a national force for education, support, empowerment, and advocacy for America's family caregivers.

I look back at what has occurred, both the good and the bad, and I look forward to the future with hope and an eye on reality.

Cindy's mom Madeleine died in 1996, and so Cindy is now a member of the "post-caregiver" contingent. Her grieving experiences during the first year after Madeleine's death gave us firsthand knowledge upon which to draw when we created a series of five bereavement articles for former caregivers.

Cindy and her husband Rich moved to California in the summer of 2001 to be closer to their daughter, son-in-law, and especially their grandchildren; but she remains on the NFCA advisory board and continues to use her wonderful graphic talent to help communicate NFCA's message. We continue to collaborate and coordinate and build our friend-ship and the good work of NFCA with the help of so many others, and the generous support of individuals, foundations, and corporations.

Steven, of course, does not get better. That is the way of MS. There is always the slow, slithering deterioration of his abilities. But I know we are lucky, that his condition could have progressed much faster than it has, and I am optimistic about our future. Steven is looking toward retirement next year unless the MS insists it be sooner. That of course will be a big change, and I know we will integrate it into our lives as we have others in the past, with the inevitable bumps along the way.

Life is about change, the ones we initiate and others that come roaring into our lives like an avalanche, unplanned and unwanted. How we deal with all of them is what matters. And so I will continue to go forth, taking the lessons I have learned to heart and using them to make a better day for Steven and myself, and hopefully for the millions of other people who are family caregivers today and the millions more that will follow us.

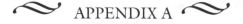

APPENDIX A

Finding Resources

The National Family Caregivers Association receives hundreds of phone calls and e-mails every month from family caregivers seeking resources, referrals, and advice. The following list includes much of the same information we provide to caregivers over the phone.

Finding Resources in Your Local Area

Find out what services and organizations are available in your local community. Even if you think you will not qualify for specific services, agencies may be able to make referrals to other organizations that may be of assistance.

- Check the county government listings in your local phone book for information on agencies:
  - ° Health and Human Services Department
  - ° Public Health Department
  - ° Social Security Administration
  - ° Mental Health Department
- Access governmental agencies and organizations online.
- Contact the social service department of your local hospital or clinic.
- Locate adult daycare centers and faith-based agencies.

- Locate the local chapter of disease groups (e.g. American Heart Association).

It is by no means certain that any of these will offer family caregiver support services; but they are a good place to check and also good sources for information about services that may directly support your loved one. State-funded services specifically for family caregivers can be found on the Web site of the Family Caregiver Alliance noted below.

Caregiver Organizations, Information, Advocacy, and Support Resources

Children of Aging Parents (CAPS)
800-227-7294
http://www.caps4caregivers.org

CAPS assists caregivers of the elderly with information and referrals, a network of support groups, and publications and programs that promote public awareness of the value and the needs of family caregivers.

Family Caregiver Alliance (FCA)
800-445-8106
e-mail: info@caregiver.org
http://www.caregiver.org

FCA is the lead agency in California's system of Caregiver Resource Centers. FCA provides support and help to family caregivers and champions their cause through education, services, research and advocacy. Services are specific to California, although information can be accessed nationally.

Family Voices, Inc.
888-835-5669
http://www.familyvoices.org

Family Voices offers information on healthcare policies relevant to special needs children in every state.

Friends' Health Connection
800-483-7436
http://www.48friend.org

Friends' Health Connection links persons with illness or disability and their family caregivers with others experiencing the same challenges.

National Alliance for Caregiving
http://www.caregiving.org

Although not an organization that helps family caregivers directly, the National Alliance for Caregiving has a Web site that helps family caregivers learn about information, videos, pamphlets, and so on that have been reviewed and approved as providing solid information.

National Family Caregivers Association
800-896-3650
http://www.thefamilycaregiver.org
e-mail: info@thefamilycaregiver.org

NFCA empowers family caregivers to develop the confidence and capabilities they need to deal with the day-to-day difficulties of their lives. Regardless of their loved one's age or diagnosis, NFCA offers a community of support, information, and education. Speaking with the authentic voice of experience, NFCA strives to break down existing barriers to the health and wellbeing of family caregivers.

Rosalynn Carter Institute for Human Development (RCI)
229-928-1234
http://www.rosalynncarter.org

RCI provides educational programs for caregivers, conducts research, and disseminates information about caregiving.

Well Spouse Association
800-838-0879
http://www.wellspouse.org
e-mail: info@wellspouse.org

Well Spouse is a national membership organization that gives support to husbands, wives, and partners of the chronically ill and/or disabled. Well Spouse has a network of support groups and also a newsletter for spouses.

Caregiver-Specific Web Sites
There are a variety of Web sites which offer information and support for family caregivers. Web sites with key information and support for family caregivers include:

Caregiver.com
800-829-2734
http://www.caregiver.com
e-mail: info@caregiver.com

Caregiver.com produces *Today's Caregiver Magazine*, the first national magazine dedicated to caregivers, the Sharing Wisdom caregivers conferences, and a Web site that includes topic-specific newsletters and online discussion lists.

CarePages
888-852-5521
http://www.carepages.com

CarePages are free, private Web pages that make it easy to reach out and receive messages of support and to stay connected to family, friends, coworkers and others who care about you and your loved one. The service is available to anyone caring for a loved one, but may be particularly helpful to those who have recently found themselves in a caregiving role.

Lotsa Helping Hands
http://www.nfca.lotsahelpinghands.com
e-mail: info@lotsahelpinghands.com

Lotsa Helping Hands is a volunteer coordination service for friends, family, colleagues, and neighbors to assist loved ones in need. It's an easy-to-use, private, group calendar specifically designed for organizing helpers, where everyone can pitch in with meal deliveries, rides, and other tasks necessary for life to run smoothly during a crisis.

Strength for Caring
866-466-3458
http://www.strengthforcaring.com

Strength for Caring is an online resource and community for family caregivers that helps them take care of their loved ones and themselves. Strength for Caring is part of the Caregiver Initiative, created by Johnson & Johnson Consumer Products Company, Division of Johnson & Johnson Consumer Companies, Inc.

Caring for Elders

Vital information and possible support services for the elderly can be obtained by contacting your local county office of senior services or elder affairs as well as your local social service department. Area adult daycare centers may also provide information on resources for the elderly in your area. These numbers can be located in the governmental pages of the phone book or through a Web search engine.

AARP
800-424-3410
http://www.aarp.org

AARP supplies information about caregiving, long-term care, and aging, including publications and audio-visual aids for caregivers.

Eldercare Locator
National Association of Area Agencies on Aging
800-677-1116
http://www.n4a.org or
http://www.eldercare.gov

Eldercare Locator provides referrals to Area Agencies on Aging via zip code locations. Family caregivers can also find information about many eldercare issues and services available in local communities.

The National Association of Professional Geriatric Care Managers
520-881-8008
http://www.caremanager.org

Geriatric care managers (GCMs) are healthcare professionals, most often social workers, who help families in dealing with the problems and challenges associated with caring for the elderly. This national organization will refer family caregivers to their state chapters, which in turn can provide the names of GCMs in your area. This information is also available online.

U.S. Administration on Aging
202-619-0724
http://www.aoa.gov

The Administration on Aging is the official federal agency dedicated to the delivery of supportive home- and community-based services to older individuals and their caregivers. The AoA Web site has a special section on family caregiving.

End-of-Life Planning, Hospice,
and Bereavement Information

Aging with Dignity
888-5-WISHES (594-7437)
http://www.agingwithdignity.org

Aging with Dignity publishes the "Five Wishes Living Will" document, a very user-friendly and comprehensive document that meets legal requirements in thirty-five states.

Caring Connections
http://www.caringinfo.org

Caring Connections provides free brochures on end-of-life topics including advance care planning, caregiving, hospice and palliative care, pain, grief and loss, and financial issues. Caring Connections also provides Advanced Directives for all states.

The Compassionate Friends
877-969-0010
http://www.compassionatefriends.org

This group offers telephone support and understanding to families who have lost a child. They maintain a resource library and have a national chapter network and newsletter.

Get Palliative Care
212-201-2670
http://www.getpalliativecare.org

Valuable information for patients and families coping with serious, complex illness including a palliative care provider directory, a definition and detailed description of palliative care, direct links to palliative care-related organizations, and more.

Hospice Foundation of America
800-854-3402
http://www.hospicefoundation.org

The National Hospice Foundation hosts an annual teleconference on issues of bereavement, and has publications on grief and bereavement.

HospiceDirectory.org
800-868-5171
http://hospicedirectory.org

Online consumer database that lists hospices in the United States, Canada, and Mexico. All hospices are listed at no cost. It is a free service that assists families and individuals in locating a hospice within their community quickly. Also provides reliable information about hospice and end-of-life care to consumers.

Health Insurance: Prescription Assistance Information
Family caregivers can contact their county or state Department of Health and Human Services for financial programs that may provide assistance for acquiring health insurance and prescription medications. Other possible financial resources may include social service agencies such as Catholic Charities, the Association of Jewish Families, and Children's Agencies. Local chapters of voluntary health agencies may also offer financial support programs and/or information on how to apply for such programs.

Benefits Check-Up
http://www.benefitscheckup.org

A service of the National Council on the Aging, Benefits Check-Up helps people over the age of fifty-five find federal, state, and local public and private programs that may pay for some of their medical care and/or prescription costs. A companion site, www.benefitscheckuprx.org, provides information about prescription medication programs.

HealthInsurance.com
800-942-9019
http://www.healthinsurance.com

This Web site provides consumers and small businesses with quotes for health insurance and may help those who have lost their health insurance find an affordable alternative.

Medicare Rights Center
888-HMO-9050
http://www.medicarerights.org

Now consumers, caregivers, and healthcare professionals across the country can access the timeliest Medicare information and resources, including state-specific information on picking the right plans, how to file an appeal, and what to do in the prescription drug coverage gap. Search within broad topics, look up basic information, or seek out specific terms.

Medicare Rx Matters
http://www.MedicareRxMatters.org

Designed to help users make decisions about the new Medicare prescription drug plan, this site has three specific portals: one for family caregivers, one for people with Medicare, and one for professionals. The Web site provides an overview, easy-to-understand steps, and information to assist users in making personal decisions about Medicare prescription drug coverage.

Medicare800-MEDICARE
http://www.medicare.gov

This is the official Web site for the Centers for Medicare and Medicaid Services (CMS), the agency responsible for Medicare Part D. Low-income subsidies are available.

Medicine Program
573-996-7300
http://www.themedicineprogram.com

This program is for persons who do not have coverage either through insurance or government subsidies for outpatient prescription drugs and for those who cannot afford to purchase medications at retail prices.

National Association of Counties
877-321-2652
https://naco.advancerx.com

The Web site list counties that have prescription assistance programs.

Partnership for Prescription Assistance
888-477-2669
www.pparx.org

The partnership is a clearinghouse of more than 475 public and private prescription assistance programs.
NeedyMeds
www.NeedyMeds.com

NeedyMeds is a free, online clearinghouse to help people who cannot afford medicine or healthcare costs. This Web site includes a wide range of information about services such as discount drug cards, Medicaid Web sites, federal poverty guidelines, and other useful information. NeedyMeds also publishes *PAP News*, a quarterly newsletter with up-to-date information about patient assistance programs (PAPs).

RxAssist
www.rxassist.org

RxAssist offers a comprehensive database of PAPs. It was established in 1997 with support from the Robert Wood

Johnson Foundation by Volunteers in Health Care, a national resource center for safety-net organizations.

RxCompare™
Email: info@maprx.info
http://www.maprx.info

RxCompare™ is a free tool developed by Medicare Access for Patients-Rx (MAPRx) to help users determine if they need to enroll in a Medicare drug plan, and, if they do, to systematically compare the drug plans where they live and select the best option for their prescription needs. RxCompare™ works in tandem with Medicare's online "Prescription Drug Plan Finder" and with information available from plans or 1-800-MEDICARE.

Together Rx Access™
www.TogetherRxAccess.com
800-250-2839

Together Rx Access™ provides a free prescription savings card for individuals who are legal residents of the United States and Puerto Rico, are not eligible for Medicare, do not have prescription drug coverage, and meet certain household income levels. The Together Rx Access™ Card was created by ten pharmaceutical companies, providing access to more than three hundred brand-name prescription and generic products.

Patient Advocacy Assistance and Programs

Patient Advocate Foundation
800-532-5274
http://www.patientadvocate.org

Patient Advocate Foundation serves as a liaison between patients and their insurer, employer, and/or creditors to resolve insurance, job retention, and/or debt crisis matters relating to a patient's condition.

Center for Patient Partnerships at the University of Wisconsin
608 265-6267
http://www.law.wisc.edu/patientadvocacy/

The center offers help in solving insurance snarls and making sense of medical bills, searching for a second opinion, and determining your eligibility for federal and state benefit programs for people with chronic or life-threatening illnesses.

Consumer Consortium on Assisted Living (CCAL)
703-533-8121
http://www.ccal.org

CCAL is a national, consumer-focused organization that is dedicated to representing the needs of residents in assisted living facilities and educating consumers, professionals, and the general public about assisted living issues. Family caregivers can request the publication *Choosing an Assisted Living Facility: Strategies for Making the Right Decision*, which provides helpful information and a concise checklist for those contemplating this next step.

National Citizens' Coalition for Nursing Home Reform
202-332-2275
http://www.nccnhr.org

This organization serves as an information clearinghouse and offers referrals nationwide for help with concerns about long-term care facilities.

Homecare Agencies, Assisted Living, and Nursing Homes

National Association for Home Care and Hospice
202-547-7424
Web site: http://www.nahc.org

This organization for home healthcare agency providers allows family caregivers to use the Internet to access a list of member agencies across the country.

New LifeStyles
800-869-9549
http://www.NewLifeStyles.com

New LifeStyles publishes regional directories of nursing homes, assisted living, and retirement communities. Call for a free copy or visit them on the Web.

Visiting Nurse Associations of America
617-737-3200
http://www.vnaa.org
vnaa@vnaa.org

VNAA promotes community based home healthcare. Family caregivers can contact them to find their local VNA.

Medical Transport and Hospitality Housing

National Association of Hospital Hospitality Houses (NAHHH)
800-542-9730
http://www.nahhh.org

NAHHH represents organizations that provide lodging and service for families receiving medical care away from home; furnishes information about hospitality homes in the caller's area; offers newsletter; and publishes an annual directory of facilities offering lodging.

National Patient Travel Center
800-296-1217
http://www.PatientTravel.org

Family caregivers can receive help locating air transportation for needy patients who need distant specialized medical evaluation, diagnosis, or treatment. The National Patient Travel Helpline is available twenty-four hours a day, seven days a week and provides referrals to all major medical transport providers in the network.

Respite Resources

Easter Seals
800-221-6827
http://www.easter-seals.org

Easter Seals provides a variety of services at four hundred sites nationwide for children and adults with disabilities, including adult daycare, in-home care, camps for special needs children, and more. Services vary by site.

Faith in Action
877-324-8411
http://www.fiavolunteers.org
info@fiavolunteers.org

Faith in Action is an interfaith volunteer caregiving program of the Robert Wood Johnson Foundation. Faith in Action makes grants to local groups representing many faiths that volunteer to care for their neighbors with long-term health needs. There are nearly one thousand interfaith volunteer caregiving programs across the country.

Family Friends
National Council on the Aging, Inc.
202-479-6672
http://www.family-friends.org

This group provides respite (and other services) by matching male and female volunteers over the age of fifty with families of children who have disabilities or chronic illness. Programs are located throughout the country.

National Adult Day Services Association, Inc.
866-890-7357
http://www.nadsa.org

This association provides information about locating adult daycare centers in your local area.

National Respite Coalition (NRC)
703-256-9578
http://www.archrespite.org/NRC.htm

NRC provides a list of states that have respite coalitions. These state coalitions then list respite services available in their state. The majority of the information is focused on helping families of children with special needs, but lately there has been an effort to enlarge their referral base to include lifespan respite information. The NRC is working to gain passage of national lifespan respite legislation.

National Respite Locator Service
800-473-1727, ext. 222
http://www.respitelocator.org/index.htm

Access a list of sites nationwide. While the vast majority focus on respite care for families of special needs children, the service now assists programs that provide respite for caregivers of adults and the elderly.

Shepherd's Centers of America
Web site: http://www.shepherdcenters.org
e-mail: staff@shepherdcenters.org

The organization provides respite care, telephone visitors, in-home visitors, nursing-home visitors, home-health aides, support groups, adult daycare, and information and referrals for accessing other services available in the community. Services vary by center.

Training for Family Caregivers

Community-based resources may offer training and classes for family caregivers. Such resources may include: your local hospital, home care agencies, Area Agency on Aging, voluntary health agencies, and county and state departments of health.

American Red Cross
202-303-4498
http://www.redcross.org

American Red Cross has developed how-to training programs for family caregivers. You will need to check with your local chapter to find out if there are classes in your area.

National Family Caregivers Association
800-896-3650
www.thefamilycaregiver.org/caregiving_resources/
workshops.cfm
infor@thefamilycaregiver.org

An educational workshop to teach family caregivers to communicate more effectively with healthcare professionals. Workshops are currently available intermittently in the community by approved trainers. Easy-to-access online and telephone programs will be available within the year.

Powerful Tools for Caregivers
www.matherflifeways.com/re_powerfultools.asp

A six-week course available in the community by licensed workshop leaders teaching family caregivers about stress reduction, finding resources, and more. An online version is also available.

Disease-Specific and Health-Related Agencies
This list was provided by the National Health Council
202-785-3910
www.nhcouncil.org
info@nhcouncil.org

Alpha-1 Foundation
888-825-7421
alphaone.org
lhall@alphaone.org

The ALS Association
818-880-9007
www.alsa.org
alsinfo@alsa-national.org

Alzheimer's Association
800-272-3900
www.alz.org
info@alz.org

American Autoimmune Related Diseases Association
800-598-4668
www.aarda.org
aarda@aol.com

American Cancer Society
800-ACS-2345 (227-2345)
www.cancer.org

American Diabetes Association
800-342-2383
www.diabetes.org
customerservice@diabetes.org

American Heart Association, Inc.
800-AHA-USA1 (242-8721)

www.americanheart.org
inquire@heart.org

American Kidney Fund
800-638-8299
www.kidneyfund.org
helpline@akfinc.org

American Liver Foundation
800-GO-LIVER (465-4837)
www.liverfoundation.org
info@liverfoundation.org

American Tinnitus Association
800-634-8978
www.ata.org
tinnitus@ata.org

Arthritis Foundation
800-283-7800
www.arthritis.org
help@arthritis.org

Asthma and Allergy Foundation
of America
800-7-ASTHMA (727-8462)
www.aafa.org
info@aafa.org

Autism Society of America
800-328-8476
www.autism-society.org

The Barth Syndrome Foundation
850-223-1128
www.barthsyndrome.org
inquiries.rd@barthsyndrome.org

CHADD (Children and Adults with Attention Deficit/ Hyperactivity Disorder)
800-233-4050
www.chadd.org
national@chadd.org

Crohn's and Colitis Foundation of America
800-932-2423
www.ccfa.org
info@ccfa.org

Easter Seals
800-221-6827
www.easter-seals.org
info@easter-seals.org

Epilepsy Foundation
800-EFA-1000 (332-1000)
www.efa.org

Huntington's Disease Society of America
800-345-HDSA (345-4372)
www.hdsa.org
hdsainfo@hdsa.org

Hydrocephalus Association
888-598-3789
www.hydroassoc.org
info@hydroassoc.org

International Pemphigus and Pemphigoid Foundation
510-527-4970
www.pemphigus.org
pemphigus@pemphigus.org

Interstitial Cystitis Association
800-HELP-ICA (435-7422)

www.ichelp.com
icamail@ichelp.org

Kidney Cancer Association
800-850-9132
www.curekidneycancer.org
office@curekidneycancer.org

The LAM Foundation
513-777-6889
www.thelamfoundation.org
lam@thelamfoundation.org

Lance Armstrong Foundation, Inc.
512-236-8820
www.laf.org

The Leukemia and Lymphoma Society
800-955-4572
www.leukemia.org
infocenter@leukemia-lymphoma.org

Lupus Foundation of America, Inc.
800-558-0121
www.lupus.org
info@lupus.org

March of Dimes Foundation
914-997-4504
www.marchofdimes.com

Mental Health America
800-969-NMHA (969-6642)
mentalhealthamerica.net

Mesothelioma Applied Research Foundation
805-563-8400

www.marf.org
info@marf.org

Myasthenia Gravis Foundation of America, Inc.
800-541-5454
www.myasthenia.org
mgfa@myasthenia.org

National Alopecia Areata Foundation
415-472-3780
www.alopeciaareata.com
info@naaf.org

National Down Syndrome Society
800-221-4602
www.ndss.org
info@ndss.org

National Eczema Association for Science and Education
800-818-7546
www.nationaleczema.org
info@nationaleczema.org

The National Foundation for Ectodermal Dysplasias
618-566-2020
www.nfed.org
info@nfed.org

National Kidney Foundation
800-622-9010
www.kidney.org
info@kidney.org

National Marfan Foundation
800-8-MARFAN (862-7326) ext.10
www.marfan.org
staff@marfan.org

National Multiple Sclerosis Society
800-FIGHT-MS
(344-4867)
www.nmss.org
info@nmss.org

National Osteoporosis Foundation
202-223-2226
www.nof.org

National Psoriasis Foundation
800-723-9166
www.psoriasis.org
getinfo@psoriasis.org

National Sleep Foundation
202-347-3471
www.sleepfoundation.org
nsf@sleepfoundation.org

Osteogenesis Imperfecta
Foundation
800-981-BONE
(981-2663)
www.oif.org
bonelink@oif.org

The Paget Foundation
800-23-PAGET
(237-2438)
www.paget.org
PagetFdn@aol.com

Parent Project Muscular Dystrophy
800-714-5437
www.parentprojectmd.org
pat@parentprojectmd.org

Prevent Blindness America
800-331-2020
www.preventblindness.org
info@preventblindness.org

RESOLVE, The National Infertility Association
888-623-0744
www.resolve.org
info@resolve.org

Restless Legs Syndrome Foundation
877-463-6757
www.rls.org
rlsfoundation@rls.org

Sjögren's Syndrome Foundation
800-4SJOGREN
(475-6473)
www.sjogrens.com
ssf@sjogrens.org

Spina Bifida Association
800-621-3141
www.sbaa.org
sbaa@sbaa.org

Tourette Syndrome Association, Inc.
888-4-TOURET
(486-8738)
http://www.tsa-usa.org

Tuberous Sclerosis Alliance
800-225-6872
http://www.tsalliance.org

Us TOO International, Inc.
800-80 US TOO

(808-7866)
www.ustoo.org
ustoo@ustoo.org

Y-ME National Breast Cancer Organization
800-221-2141
www.y-me.org
help@y-me.org

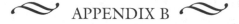

APPENDIX B

Family Caregiving and Public Policy

Family Caregiving and Public Policy Principles for Change*

Caregiving has always been a universal experience in society affecting people of all races, ethnicities, lifestyles, and income levels, but in our time family caregiving has become more than an act of love and familial responsibility. It has become an essential element of our health and long-term care system. This is so for a number of reasons:

- Historically caregiving was short-lived. Most people died from infectious diseases until the advent of antibiotics in the twentieth century. The average lifespan in 1900 was forty-seven. Today it is in the mid-70s, and the majority of people die from the consequences of a chronic condition. This means caregiving situations typically last years or decades—or, in some cases, such as when children are born with congenital abnormalities or developmental disabilities, an entire lifetime.

- Institutionalization of individuals with chronic or disabling conditions has given way to a growing movement toward mainstreaming and community living. This movement has now become the law of the land with the handing down of the Supreme Court's *Olmstead* decision.

- In the midst of these changes, major demographic trends are also having an impact on family caregiving.
- Family members no longer live in close proximity to the extent they did in the past. Long-distance caregiving is a result of our enhanced mobility and changing social order.
- Women have traditionally played the role of family caregiver, but in this era when women make up almost half the labor force, they are less available to take on the role of family caregiver.

Add to these changes the fact that America is currently facing an ever-growing healthcare-worker shortage at the same time that health and long-term care costs continue to rise. As a result of cost containment policies and practices, people with health needs are being discharged from hospitals or other acute-care settings with more complex care needs and curtailed homecare services, which means more responsibility for families, who are inadequately prepared and trained.

It is clear that given these circumstances American healthcare is now on a collision course with the day-to-day reality of families coping with chronic conditions. Without attention to this situation, the $257 billion in unpaid supportive services provided by the more than 25 million family caregivers[1]—an amount comparable to Medicare spending in 2002 and exceeding Medicaid spending in the same year[2]— may well be jeopardized as these same family caregivers suffer from physical, emotional, and financial problems that impede their ability to give care now and support their own care needs in the future. As this pattern plays itself out, the quality of care provided to individuals with disabling or chronic conditions or the frail elderly will diminish and the costs to the nation's healthcare system skyrocket.

Now more than ever, the United States needs to develop responsible social policy to address the needs of caregiving families who have unwittingly taken on the dual jobs of healthcare and social-service provider. The following principles apply to caregivers in all situations, although how they would be implemented would vary by setting.

*This Statement of Principles was developed in 2003 and publicly presented at the first National Town Hall Meeting on family caregiving in February 2004 on Capitol Hill, Washington, DC. Although some of the statistics cited have changed since the preparation of these principles, the document is as valid today as when it was first released.

The principles were developed by: Lynn Friss Feinberg, National Center on Caregiving/Family Caregiver Alliance; Jane Horvath, Health Policy Analyst; Gail Hunt and Les Plooster, National Alliance for Caregiving; Jill Kagan, National Respite Coalition; Carol Levine, Families and Healthcare Project, United Hospital Fund; Joanne Lynn, MD, Americans for Better Care of the Dying; Suzanne Mintz, National Family Caregivers Association; Anne Wilkinson, Rand Corporation.

Principle One

Family caregiving concerns must be a central component of healthcare, long-term care, and social-service policymaking.

- Family caregivers provide approximately 80 percent of all long-term services and support for family members and friends across the lifespan.[3, 4]
- Services provided each year by family caregivers are conservatively worth $257 billion, more than double the annual spending on home care and nursing-home care combined, and comparable to 20 percent of all healthcare spending.[5]
- Family caregivers put their own health and wellbeing at risk in the service of their loved ones as they simultaneously save the healthcare system significant amounts of money.[6, 7]

Despite the wealth of services they provide, and in spite of their staggering numbers, family caregivers continue to be the most neglected group of the health and long-term care system. In return for family caregivers' contributions to the public good, society, through its public and private sectors, must support caregivers through well-designed policies, programs, and practices.

Principle Two

Family caregivers must be protected against the financial, physical, and emotional consequences of caregiving that can put their own health and wellbeing in jeopardy.

- Among their many roles, family caregivers are integral but unpaid partners in the healthcare system. As such, they provide care at significant costs to themselves.
- Out-of-pocket medical expenses for a family that has a loved one with a disabling or chronic condition who needs help with activities of daily living (eating, toileting, etc.) are more than 2.5 times greater than for a family without a family member with a disabling or chronic condition (11.2% of income compared to 4.1%).[8]
- The majority of caregivers are employed and many are forced to make changes at work to accommodate caregiving. Over the course of a caregiving "career," family caregivers providing intense personal care can lose as much as $659,000 in wages, pensions, and Social Security.[9]
- Family caregivers who provide care thirty-six or more hours weekly are more likely than non-caregivers to experience symptoms of depression or anxiety. For spouses the rate is six times higher; for those caring for a parent the rate is twice as high.[10]
- Caregivers use prescription drugs for depression, anxiety, and insomnia two to three times as often as the rest of the population.[11]
- The stress of intense family caregiving for persons with dementia has been shown to impact a person's immune system both in terms of increased chances of

developing a chronic illness and in significantly slowing wound healing.[12, 13]

Principle Three

Family caregivers must have access to affordable, readily
available, high-quality respite care as a key component of the
supportive-services network.

- Respite, often the most frequently requested family
  support service,[14] provides caregivers with occasional
  relief necessary to sustain their own health or attend
  to other family members. In emergency situations, a
  temporary haven to ensure the safety of the person for
  whom they provide care and provide the care receiver
  with a quality experience as well becomes an absolute
  necessity.
- Without respite, not only can families suffer economi-
  cally and emotionally, caregivers themselves may face
  serious health and social risks as a result of stress associated with continuous caregiving.[15]
- Respite has been shown to help sustain family stability,
  avoid out-of-home placements, and reduce the likelihood of abuse and neglect.[16] New preliminary data
  from an outcome-based evaluation pilot study show
  that respite may also reduce the likelihood of divorce
  and help sustain marriages.[17]
- Respite, however, remains in short supply for all age
  groups, or is inaccessible to the family because of
  eligibility requirements, geographic barriers, cost,
  or the lack of culturally sensitive programs. Thus
  lifespan systems need to be in place to identify and
  coordinate federal, state, and community-based respite resources and funding streams across ages, disabilities, and family circumstances; provide easy access to an array of affordable, quality, respite services; to ensure flexibility to meet diverse needs; to
  fill gaps and address barriers in existing services; and

to assist family caregivers with locating, training, and paying for respite.

Principle Four

Family caregivers must be supported by family-friendly policies in the workplace to meet their caregiving responsibilities. Examples of family-friendly workplace policies include: flextime; work-at-home options; job-sharing; counseling; dependent care accounts; information and referral to community services; employer-paid services of a care manager and more.

- Currently, only large Fortune 500 companies tend to have programs to support family caregivers—and then only for those caregiving for elderly relatives. Few small and mid-sized businesses—where most Americans work—have programs supporting family caregivers and are increasingly cutting paid health benefits as well. As a result, most family caregivers struggle to balance work and family responsibilities.
- Forty-two percent of parents of children with special needs lack basic workplace supports, such as paid sick leave and vacation time.[18]
- Family caregivers are doubly penalized when they temporarily leave the workforce for caregiving. Not only may they lose actual pay, but they also lose social security credits, which can impact their own ability to care for themselves in the future.

Principle Five

Family caregivers must have appropriate, timely, and ongoing education and training to successfully meet their caregiving responsibilities and to be advocates for their loved ones across care settings.

- Family caregiving is a complex responsibility involving emotional support, household management, medical care, dealing with a variety of governmental and other agencies, and decision making. Yet family caregivers consistently report that they were "not prepared" for these roles. This lack of training occurs throughout the caregiving experience, but is most apparent when care recipients are discharged from hospitals or short-term nursing-home stays after an illness or accident. One national survey found that 43 percent of caregivers performed at least one medical task, defined as bandaging and wound care, operating medical equipment, or managing a medication regimen.[19] Yet formal instruction is sporadic and inadequate. Families are expected to perform "skilled" nursing care, but without the training that professionals must receive.

- Family caregivers' needs for information and training change throughout the course of their loved one's illness. They must have opportunities to learn new skills as they become necessary, access new resources, and learn about options for care as the situation changes. Families need honest information about the financial, social, and health-related consequences of various arrangements for care, and they must share in the decision making about care arrangements.

- Professionals must provide information in understandable, nonjudgmental, and culturally competent ways that reflect sensitivity to the caregiver's emotional involvement with the care recipient. Policy makers should support programs that bring family caregivers and professionals together to further collaboration.[20]

Principle Six

Family caregivers and their loved ones must have affordable, readily available, high-quality, comprehensive services that are coordinated across all care settings.

- People who need the assistance of family caregivers typically have complex, chronic medical conditions and functional limitations. As a result, they require services from many parts of the medical and long-term care systems. Unfortunately, coordination of information and services within each system and between these systems rarely occurs.

- Use of community services increases with level of disability as well as with age. Thirteen percent of people older than eighty-five use community services (home-delivered meals, transportation, care management, etc.) compared to only 1 percent of persons aged fifty to sixty-four. Case-management services play an important role in linking persons with available services as well as managing public expenditures for long-term services.[21]

- Thirty-two percent of people with serious chronic conditions see four or more different physicians in a year. Medicare beneficiaries with five or more conditions see an average of fourteen different physicians in a year.[22]

- In 2000, 50 percent of caregivers reported that different providers gave different diagnoses for the same set of symptoms and 62 percent reported that different providers gave other conflicting information. Another recent survey found that 44 percent of physicians believe poor care coordination leads to unnecessary hospitalization, and 24 percent stated poor care coordination can lead to otherwise unnecessary nursing-home stays.[23]

- It is in this environment that caregivers must take on the complicated and difficult role of care coordinator—ensuring that treatments prescribed by different providers do not conflict and ensuring that important medical and functional information travels across providers, settings, and over time. Care coordination (within the medical system and across medical and supportive-service systems) is not common in healthcare today.[24] Lack of coordination, resulting in poor health outcomes, can drive inappropriate and potentially unnecessary spending.

Principle Seven

Family caregivers and their loved ones must be assured of an affordable, well-qualified, and sustainable healthcare workforce across all care settings.

- Millions of family caregivers and their loved ones require medical and non-medical assistance from direct-care workers, either at home or in institutional settings. Currently, there is a growing shortage of these paraprofessional and professional workers that is impacting the quality and continuity of care. The problem is projected to get worse as the Baby Boom Generation ages.[25]
- A shortage of well-qualified, reliable, and affordable healthcare workers has a direct impact on the health and safety of persons with chronic conditions or disabilities. It also has a direct impact on the health and wellbeing of family caregivers who must pick up the extra workload, much of which requires training and support they do not have, and which adds to their caregiving burden.[28]

Principle Eight

Family caregivers must have access to regular comprehensive assessments of their caregiving situation to determine what assistance they may require.

- Social service and healthcare providers cannot assume that family members can always provide care for a frail elder or person with disabilities.
- Family caregivers should be considered an integral part of the long-term care system, as individuals with rights to their own support and assessments of their own needs.

- An assessment of the family caregiver's strengths, needs, and preferences constitutes the foundation for developing appropriate and quality long-term care.[29]
- The availability of family members or others to provide uncompensated care should not be considered in allocating long-term care benefits (as in the Medicaid program).

Endnotes

1. Arno, P.S. (February 24, 2002). *Economic Value of Informal Caregiving*. Orlando, FL: Annual Meeting of the American Association of Geriatric Psychiatry.
2. MedPAC. (2002). *Report to the Congress: Assessing Medicare Benefits*. Washington, DC: MedPAC.
3. US General Accounting Office. (1994). *Long-Term Care: Diverse, Growing Population Includes Millions of Americans of All Ages* (GAO/HEHS 95-26). Washington, DC: GAO.
4. Agency for Healthcare Research and Quality (2000). *The Characteristics of Long-Term Care Users*. Silver Spring, MD: AHRQ.
5. Arno, P. S. (February 24, 2002). *Economic Value of Informal Caregiving*. Orlando, FL: Annual Meeting of the American Association of Geriatric Psychiatry.
6. MacCallum, R., et al. (2003). Chronic Stress and Age-Related Increases in the Proinflammatory IL–6. *Proceedings of the National Academy of Science, 100*(15), 9090 – 9095.
7. Schulz R, & Beach, S.R. (1999). Caregiving as a risk factor for mortality: The caregiver health effects study. *JAMA, 282*, 2215-2219.
8. Altman, Cooper, & Cunningham. (1999). The Case of Disability in the Family: Impact on Health Care Utilization and Expenditures for Non-disabled Members. *Milbank Quarterly*, 77 (1), 39 – 75.
9. National Alliance for Caregiving and Brandeis University National Center on Women and Aging (1999). *The MetLife Juggling Act Study: Balancing Caregiving with Work and the Costs Involved*. Westport, CT: MetLife Mature Market Institute.
10. Cannuscio, C.C., C Jones, C., Kawachi, I., Colditz, G.A., Berkman, L., & Rimm, E. (2002). Reverberation of family illness: A longitudinal assessment of informal caregiver and mental health status in the nurses' health study. *American Journal of Public Health, 92*, 305-1311.
11. George, L.K., & Gwyther, L.P. (1986). Caregiver Well-Being:

A Multidimensional Examination of Family Caregivers of Demented Adults. *The Gerontologist*, 26(2), 253-260. As cited by Scharlach, A.E., Lowe, B.F., and Schneider, E.L. (1991). *Elder Care and the Work Force: Blueprint for Action*. Ontario, Canada: Lexington Books.

12. Kiecolt-Glaser, J., Trask, O.J., Speicher, J.R., & Glaser, R. (1995). Slowing of Wound Healing by Psychological Distress. *The Lancet*, 346, 1194-1196.

13. Schulz, R. & Beach, S. R. (1999). Caregiving as a Risk Factor for Mortality: The Caregiver Health Effects Study. *Journal of the American Medical Association*, 282(23).

14. National Alliance for Caregiving & AARP (1997). *Family Caregiving in the U.S.: Findings From a National Survey*. Bethesda, MD: Authors, 1997.

15. 1) Abelson, A.G. (1999). Economic Consequences and Lack of Respite Care. *Psychological Reports*, 85, 880-882; 2) Sherman, B.R. (1995). Impact of home-based respite care on families of children with chronic illnesses. *Children's Health Care*, 24(1), 33-45; 3) Theis, S.L., Moss, J.H. & Pearson, M.A. (1994). Respite for caregivers: An evaluation study. *Journal of Community Health Nursing*, 11(1), 31-34; and 4) Zarit, S.H., Parris Stephens, M.S., Townsend, A., & Greene, R. (1998). Stress reduction for family caregivers: Effect of adult day care use. *The Journal of Gerontology*, 53B(5), S267-S277.

16. 1) ARCH National Respite Network and Resource Center (2002). *Annotated Bibliography of Respite and Crisis Care Studies: Second Edition*. Chapel Hill, NC: ARCH National Respite Network and Resource Center; 2) Cohen, S. & Warren, R. (1985). *Respite Care: Principles, Programs, and Polices*. Austin, TX: PRO-ED; 3) Wade, C., Kirk, R., Edgar, M., & Baker, L. (2003). *Outcome Evaluation: Phase II Results*. Chapel Hill, NC: ARCH National Resource Center for Respite and Crisis Care.

17. Wade, C., Kirk, R., Edgar, M., & Baker, L. (2003). *Outcome Evaluation: Phase II Results*. Chapel Hill, NC: ARCH National Resource Center for Respite and Crisis Care.

18. Heyman, J. (2000). *The Widening Gap*. New York: Basic Books.

19. Donelan, K., et al. (2002). Challenged To Care: Informal Caregivers in a Changing Health System. *Health Affairs,* July/August 2002, 222-231.

20. Levine, C. (1998). Rough Crossings: Family Caregivers' Odysseys through the Health Care System. New York: United Hospital Fund.

21. AARP (2003). *Beyond 50 2003 - A Report to the Nation on Independent Living and Disability*. Washington, DC: AARP.

22. *Op. cit.*
23. *Op. cit.*
24. DeJonge, E. & Leff, B. (2003, August 7). A Real Medicare Remedy. *Washington Post*, p. A21.
25. ASPE, CMS, HRSA, DOL Office of the Assistant Secretary for Policy; BLS & ETA (2003). *Future Supply of Long-term Care Workers in Relation to the Aging Baby Boom Generation: Report to Congress.* Washington, DC: ASPE.
26. Donelan, K., et al. (2002). Challenged To Care: Informal Caregivers in a Changing Health Care System. *Health Affairs*, July/August 2002, 222-231.
27. Feinberg, L.F. (in press). The state of the art of caregiver assessment. *Generations.*
28. Feinberg, L.F., Newman, S.L. & Van Steenberg, C. (2002). *Family Caregiver Support: Policies, Perceptions and Practices in 10 States Since Passage of the National Family Caregiver Support Program.* San Francisco: Family Caregiver Alliance.
29. Gaugler, J.E., Kane, R.A. & Langlois, J. (2000). Assessment of family caregivers of older adults. In R.L. and R.A.Kane, eds. *Assessing Older Persons: Measures, Meaning and Practical Applications.* New York: Oxford University Press.

Summary of Caregiving Legislation in 110th Congress January–June 2007

Many bills have been introduced in Congress related to family caregiving. Information on the bills is presented below in the following categories: Respite; Tax Bills; Social Security/Medicare/Medicaid Enhancements; Family Leave Enhancements; and Other Legislation.

Bill Number and Title	Sponsors	Status
Alzheimer's Caregivers		
H.R. 1032 Alzheimer's Treatment and Caregiver Support Act	Rep. Maxine Waters (D-CA); forty cosponsors	Referred to House Committee on Energy and Commerce on February 13, 2007.
How this helps family caregivers: Authorizes "such sums as may be necessary" for FY08–FY13 for expanded Health and Human Services (HHS) grants for public and nonprofit programs that combine Alzheimer's treatment with additional training and support services for family caregivers of Alzheimer's patients; at least 10 percent of the grants would have to be directed to healthcare facilities that primarily care for medically underserved communities.		
S. 898, H.R. 1560 Alzheimer's Breakthrough Act of 2007	Sen. Barbara Mikulski (D-MD); twenty-one cosponsors	Referred to the Senate Committee on Health, Education, Labor, and Pensions on March 15, 2007.
	Rep. Edward Markey (D-MA); thirty-nine cosponsors	Referred to the House Committee on Energy and Commerce on March 19, 2007.
How this helps family caregivers: The bill amends the Public Health Service Act to fund breakthroughs in Alzheimer's disease research while providing more help to caregivers and increasing public education about prevention. Among other things, it also requires the Director of the National Institute on Aging to conduct, or award grants for, clinical, social, and behavioral research related to interventions designed to help caregivers of patients with Alzheimer's disease and related disorders and improve patient outcomes.		

Bill Number and Title	Sponsors	Status
Tax Bills		
S. 614 Middle Class Opportunity Act of 2007	Sen. Charles Schumer (D-NY); eleven cosponsors	Referred to the Senate Committee on Finance on February 15, 2007.
How this helps family caregivers: Amends the Internal Revenue Code to expand eligibility for the dependent-care tax credit and allow such credit for expenses to care for parents and grandparents who do not reside with the taxpayer. Currently, a caregiver's mother or father must be living with them in order to claim the credit.		
S. 897, H.R. 1807 Alzheimer's Family Assistance Act of 2007	Sen. Barbara Mikulski (D-MD); eighteen cosponsors Rep. Eddie Bernice Johnson (D-TX); no cosponsors	Referred to Senate Committee on Finance on March 15, 2007. Referred to House Committee on Ways and Means on March 29, 2007.
How this helps family caregivers: Amends the Internal Revenue Code to: (1) allow a phased-in tax credit ($1,000 in 2007 increasing by $500 each year until allowing $3,000 in 2011) for family caregivers of spouses and dependents who have long-term care needs; (2) allow a tax deduction for long-term care insurance premiums; and (3) apply certain consumer protection standards to long-term care insurance contracts.		
H.R. 1911 Tax Relief for Working Caregivers Act of 2007	Rep. Joe Donnelly (D-IN); four cosponsors	Referred to House Committee on Ways and Means on April 18, 2007.
How this helps family caregivers: Amends the Internal Revenue Code to expand eligibility for the dependent-care tax credit to allow such credit for expenses to care for parents and grandparents who do not reside with the taxpayer and who are physically or mentally incapable of caring for himself or herself. Currently, a caregiver's mother or father must be living with them in order to claim the credit.		
S. 158 Access to Affordable Health Care Act	Sen. Susan Collins (R-ME); one cosponsor	Referred to Senate Committee on Finance on January 4, 2007.

con't. on page 188

Bill Number and Title	Sponsors	Status
con't. from page 187	**Tax Bills**	

How this helps family caregivers: Wide-ranging healthcare bill whose provisions include: (1) tax credits to small businesses for qualified employee health insurance expenses; (2) tax credits for qualified health insurance; (3) deductions for long-term care insurance premiums; and (4) tax credits for individuals with long-term care needs (recipients only). This graduated tax credit begins at $1,000 in FY05 and would rise yearly by $500 increments until it reaches its ceiling of $3,000 in FY09 and beyond.

Social Security / Medicare / Medicaid Enhancements*		
H.R. 1161 Social Security Caregiver Credit Act of 2007	Rep. Nita Lowey (D-NY); no cosponsors	Referred to the House Committee on Ways and Means on February 16, 2007.

How this helps family caregivers: Would allow unpaid family caregivers to claim Social Security benefits, payable under the old age, survivors, and disability insurance, as if they had worked for a wage (according to a specified formula) during each month they were engaged for at least eighty hours in providing care to a dependent relative, for up to five years of such service.

S. 1340, H.R. 2244 Geriatric Assessment and Chronic Care Coordination Act of 2007	Sen. Blanche Lincoln (D-AR); nine cosponsors	Introduced on May 9, 2007 in the Senate. Will be referred to Senate Finance Committee soon.
	Rep. Gene Green (D-TX); three cosponsors	Introduced on May 9, 2007 in the House. Will be referred to the Committees on Ways and Means, and Energy and Commerce soon.

How this helps family caregivers: The bill authorizes coverage of geriatric assessments and chronic-care coordination services in the Medicare fee-for-service program for certain high-cost beneficiaries who have either multiple chronic conditions *or* dementia and

Bill Number and Title	Sponsors	Status
Medicare / Medicaid Enhancements*		

at least one chronic condition. Chronic care involves the treatment of multiple health conditions that limit the patient. The current Medicare program penalizes physicians for coordinating healthcare because they are not paid for these services, resulting with episodic care to generate more visits. Under this new benefit, Medicare would pay physicians and other eligible providers to provide geriatric assessments and coordinate chronic care.

A geriatric assessment is a comprehensive review of an individual's medical condition, functional and cognitive capacity, as well as caregiver, environmental, and psychosocial needs. A written care plan will identify problems, therapies, and assignments for future actions. Individuals who have been assessed and deemed likely to benefit from care coordination services may elect to use this benefit and choose a chronic-care manager. Chronic-care managers may include Medicare-approved physicians, physician assistants, nurse practitioners, clinical nurse specialists, and/or clinical social workers. Chronic-care services may include: (1) development/implementation of a care plan coordinated with physicians, medical personnel, and agencies; (2) use of evidence-based medicine and clinical-decision support for providers; (3) use of health information technology to track patients' health status; (4) education and encouragement so patients can manage their own health; (5) medication monitoring and management; (6) telephone consultations, including twenty-four-hour availability; (7) education and inclusion of caregivers into the planning process; (8) management of transitions among healthcare professionals and settings of care; and (9) referrals to community services and hospice services.

| S. 799, H.R. 1621 Community Choice Act of 2007 | Sen. Tom Harkin (D-IA); fourteen cosponsors | Referred to Senate Committee on Finance on March 7, 2007. |
| | Rep. Danny Davis (D-IL); eighteen cosponsors | Referred to House Committee on Energy and Commerce on March 21, 2007. |

con't. on page 190

Bill Number and Title	Sponsors	Status
Medicare / Medicaid Enhancements*		
How this helps family caregivers: The bill would increase access to community-based services and other supports for Americans with disabilities and older Americans by requiring state Medicaid plans to cover such attendant services and supports. It would give individuals who are eligible for nursing-home services or other institutional care equal access to community-based services and supports. The legislation also provides enhanced federal-matching funds to help states develop their long-term care infrastructure and grant funds to help states increase their ability to provide home- and community-based services.		
* Note: The Medicare program does not cover most types of long-term assistance given by family caregivers at home. Medicare does provide up to thirty-five hours per week of skilled nursing care in the home, but the program does not help to pay for associated "custodial care" expenses, such as helping an incapacitated relative to shop, eat, clean, bathe, and dress. Medicare also does not cover most types of training to help caregivers learn how best to look after their families. The bills in this section address some of Medicare's shortcomings in these areas.		
Family Leave Enhancements		
S. 910, H.R. 1542 Healthy Families Act	Sen. Edward Kennedy (D-MA); twenty-two cosponsors	Referred to the Committee on Health, Education, Labor and Pensions on March 15, 2007.
	Rep. Rosa DeLauro (D-CT); forty-one cosponsors	Referred to the Committees on Education and Labor, Oversight and Government Reform, and House Administration on March 15, 2007.
How this helps family caregivers: Provides paid sick leave to employees "to ensure that Americans can address their own health needs and the health needs of their families." Specifically, the Act mandates that certain employers with at least fifteen employees provide a minimum paid sick leave of seven days annually for those who work at least thirty hours per week, as well as a prorated amount for those who work twenty to thirty hours per week, and notably allows employees to use such leave to meet their own *or* their families' medical needs.		

Bill Number and Title	Sponsors	Status
Family Leave Enhancements		
H.R. 1369 Family and Medical Leave Expansion Act	Rep. Carolyn Maloney (D-NY); one cosponsor	Referred to the House Committees on Education and the Workforce, Oversight and Government Reform, and House Administration on March 7, 2007.

How this helps family caregivers: (1) amends the Family and Medical Leave Act to enable the secretary of labor to authorize five-year grants to a state or local government to replace lost wages for individuals caring for a newly born or adopted child or taking care of "other family caregiving needs;" (2) authorizes $400 million in FY07 for the grants.

H.R. 2392 Family and Work-place Balancing Act of 2007	Rep. Lynn Woosley (D-CA); sixty-one cosponsors	Referred to the House Administration, House Armed Services, House Education and Labor, House Financial Services, House Oversight and Government Reform on May 17, 2007.

How this helps family caregivers: The bill aims to improve the lives of working families by providing family and medical-need assistance, child-care assistance, in-school and after-school assistance, family-care assistance, and encouraging the establishment of family-friendly workplaces. The bill, ambitious in scope, makes grants to eligible entities to assist families by providing wage replacement for individuals who are responding to family caregiving needs. For the wage replacements, $400,000,000 is authorized to be appropriated for FY08 and such sums as may be necessary for each of fiscal years 2009 though 2013. The bill also supports family child-care providers for young children, including those with disabilities, through support networks and programs. For the child-care programs, $500,000,000 is authorized to be appropriated for each of the fiscal years 2008, 2009, and 2010.

Bill Number and Title	Sponsors	Status
Family Leave Enhancements		
S. 1681 The Family Leave Insurance Act of 2007	Sen. Chris Dodd (D-CT); three cosponsors	Referred to the Senate Finance Committee on June 21, 2007.
How this helps family caregivers: Provides up to eight weeks of paid leave over a twelve-month period to workers needing time off owing to the birth or adoption of a child; to care for a child, spouse, or parent with serious illness; or to care for their own serious illness. Employees will have had to work for the same employer and pay insurance premiums for twelve months to receive the benefits. To fulfill this Act, a Family Leave Insurance Fund will be created. Employees, employers, and the federal government will share the costs of providing compensation during these times of need.		
Other Legislation		
S. 1065 Heroes at Home Act of 2007	Sen. Hilary Clinton (D-NY); eight cosponsors	Referred to the Committee on Armed Services on March 29, 2007.
How this helps family caregivers: Requires the secretary of Veterans Affairs to establish a program on training and certification of family caregivers of veterans and members of the armed forces with traumatic brain injury as personal-care attendants. The cost of training is borne by the secretary of Veterans Affairs. In addition, a family caregiver of a veteran or member of the Armed Forces who receives certification as a personal-care attendant would be eligible for compensation from the Department of Veterans Affairs for care provided to such veteran or member.		

Healthcare

Your Loved One's Health Information: Don't Leave Home Without It
by Sandy Padwo Rogers

No one can forget watching in horror as residents of New Orleans fled their homes in the wake of Hurricane Katrina. Thousands escaped with their lives but lost everything else. For those of us who witnessed the devastation, it was a solemn reminder of how quickly lives can change. The victims of this deadly hurricane, as well as the victims of other natural disasters, lost so much more than their homes and their other material possessions. They lost irreplaceable family treasures, crucial personal paperwork, and their complete medical histories.

It shouldn't take a natural disaster to get all of us to think about how difficult it would be to start from scratch, especially when it comes to our medical care. Just think about how many times you have had to sit in a doctor's office and recite your loved one's medical history. As a family caregiver, you serve as the care coordinator, keeping track of doctor visits, medications, tests; and therapies; most likely, you are the person each healthcare provider turns to for updates and progress reports regarding your loved one's condition. With that in mind, most of us don't normally walk around with our loved one's medical information in our pocket. Our files are scattered about—at home, at work, at the doctor's office. After all, we assume that our healthcare providers will always be there to help us re-create any information we misplace or forget. In the case of Hurricane Katrina and other natural disasters, however, many patients and their family caregivers found themselves with no paperwork, no medications, and no doctor's office or hospital to call to re-create crucial health information.

Ever since September 11, 2001, we have been hearing about emergency preparedness. The truth of the matter is that it shouldn't take a national disaster—either man-made or natural—to remind us to get our affairs—especially our medical affairs—in order. You can take a proactive role in helping your loved one and yourself by putting together a personal health record.

What Is a Personal Health Record?

Spend any time online researching medical records and you will quickly find that there is a difference between a health (or medical) record and a personal health record (PHR). Each time your loved one visits a physician's office, undergoes a procedure, or requires hospitalization, a health (or medical) record is created by the doctor, healthcare facility, or hospital. The content of this record varies depending on the services received. Most health records include: a medical history, including past surgeries and illnesses; progress notes; medication lists; test results; lab reports; physician orders; and so on. These records are maintained by the healthcare provider, although you do have the right to obtain copies upon request. A personal health record (PHR), on the other hand, is maintained by the patient and his/her family. It includes copies of all your loved one's various healthcare providers' records, along with basic health information that you and your loved one compile together.

"There are a lot of ways of looking at what a personal health record is," says Andrew Barbash, MD, a practicing neurologist in Maryland and CEO of Apractis LLC, a personal health information service. "Most people think that a personal health record is just a compilation of provider records. It is not. A personal health record is a tailored set of information that the patient and the family caregiver play an active role in creating."

The American Health Information Management Association (AHIMA), a national, nonprofit, professional association dedicated to the effective management of personal health information, defines a personal health record (PHR) as: "A universally available, lifelong resource of health information needed by individuals to make health decisions. Individuals own and manage the information in the PHR, which comes from healthcare providers and the individual. The PHR is maintained in a secure and private environment, with the individual determining rights of access. The PHR is separate from and does not replace the legal record of any provider."

The key to the PHR is *you*, the family caregiver. Unlike the health records that your loved one's doctors create, you play an active role in the creation of, the control over, and the access to your loved one's PHR. Taking ownership of his/her health information will not only make your life easier during the next doctor's visit, it will empower you to play a larger role in your loved one's healthcare.

Why Do You Need a PHR?

A PHR is valuable beyond emergency situations. Take a moment to think about how many healthcare providers your loved one sees on a regular basis. Each of these providers keeps his/her own set of medical records on your loved one's care, but those records are specific to that particular physician. Your loved one's doctors don't share this information among themselves. Each may not be aware what the other has prescribed or recommended. As the family caregiver, you are the single depository for all the disparate pieces, and only you can ensure that all of the providers involved know the "big picture." Now think about how much easier this role would be if you had one place where you kept all the information that is generated regarding your loved one's care. "By having information available in a form that makes it easy to share with healthcare providers, you have something that is very valuable to them," says John Boden, founder of Life Ledger, an Internet-based service that provides online storage for medical, legal, and financial documents for seniors. "If you want to be seen as part of the solution by the healthcare team, you need to be prepared with the information that will help them do their job, and you need to communicate this information in as easy a way as possible. " That's where the PHR comes into play.

What Information Belongs in a PHR?

Physician and hospital records, lab reports, and test results are all just one small part of a personal health record. AHIMA has put together a comprehensive list of information that you should be sure to include in any personal health record. This is an extensive list, and it would be easy to feel overwhelmed after reading it. While a complete PHR should include as much of the information listed below as possible, the key is to put together *something*, even if your record contains only a few of the items listed.

According to AHIMA, a PHR should contain:

- Personal identification, including name, birth date, and social security number. (*There is a great deal of debate about the advisability of including your social security number. This decision is an individual one and should be made only after considering how secure the PHR will be.*)
- People to contact in case of emergency
- Names, addresses, and phone numbers of your physician, dentist, and other specialists
- Health insurance information
- Living wills and advance directives
- Organ donor authorization
- A list and dates of significant illnesses and surgeries
- Current medications and dosages
- Immunizations and their dates
- Allergies

- Important events, dates, and hereditary conditions in your family history
- A recent physical examination
- Opinions of specialists
- Important test results
- Eye and dental records
- Correspondence between you and your provider(s)
- Permission forms for release of information for office visits, operations, and other medical procedures
- Any information you want to include about your health—such as exercise regime, any herbal medications you take, and any counseling you receive

Requesting Your Loved One's Health Information

The first step in putting together a PHR for your loved one is to gather the medical records from his/her various providers. The vast majority of healthcare providers still keep their medical records the old-fashioned way: in paper form. A very small percentage of providers are beginning to keep their records electronically, although it is estimated that it will be a decade or more before electronic medical records become the norm. While the physician or healthcare facility maintains these records, you have a legal right to obtain copies.

The Health Insurance Portability and Accountability Act (HIPAA) establishes the patient's right to privacy with regard to personal health information. Under HIPAA, patients have the right to request copies of their health information from their healthcare providers and these copies must be furnished within sixty days of the request. Individuals may designate others—in this case, you, the family caregiver—to have access as well. For more information on rights and protections under the federal health information privacy law, go to www.hhs.gov/ocr/hipaa/ or call toll-free 866-627-7748.

Ensuring your ability to access your care recipient's information is simple enough to accomplish. First, identify the healthcare providers from whom you need to receive information. Next, a written authorization form should be filled out and signed by your loved one. This authorization should include specific language that gives the healthcare provider permission to release to you, and/or another individual your loved one designates, any and all information regarding your loved one's treatment and care. If you have been given power of attorney for your care recipient, then *you* may be able to provide this authorization to the healthcare provider.

Keep in mind that while you have legal rights regarding your ability to obtain copies of your loved one's medical records, healthcare providers have a legal right to charge you for these copies. These charges can vary by state—and can be as high as $1 or more, per page—so it is important to be familiar with your state's law regarding the reasonable fees that can be charged for the copying and mailing of records.

Maintaining a PHR

Once you have collected the initial set of information from your loved one's healthcare providers, it is critical that you remember to update this information with each new healthcare encounter. Therein lies the daunting part of the PHR process. "It's important to collect the newest pages of the medical record as soon as they are created," says Megan Mok, president and founder of PeopleChart, a medical-record service provider that specializes in the collection, organization, and maintenance of personal health records. The prospect of having to follow up each doctor or hospital visit with a request for the newest medical records is more than some people can contemplate. When it comes time to provide this information to a physician or hospital, however, the PHR is only beneficial if it is current. "Providers use this clinical information as the basis for their future treatment decisions," says Mok. Therefore, it is critical that you keep the information updated with each new medical visit. The easiest way to do this is to request a copy before leaving the doctor's office. Since out of sight is out of mind, most of us are likely to forget to follow up afterwards.

There are a number of ways to maintain a PHR and a number of commercial services that will help you do so. The decision about which method to utilize is a very personal one, and should be made only after evaluating your needs, your comfort level with the various storage mechanisms available to you, and when and how this information may be utilized. "It's very important that before you worry about the product you will use to maintain your PHR, you take a step backward and ask a few basic questions," advises Dr. Barbash.

It may be helpful to discuss the following with your loved one:

- How comfortable are you with requesting health records personally and keeping track of doctors?
- Are you organized enough to maintain your files yourself or do you need assistance?
- How will you be using this information and who may need to see it?
- If you choose to keep your PHR online or to utilize a disk or other portable device, will the healthcare providers who may be retrieving this information have access to the technology needed to do so?
- Does your loved one's information need to be readily available to any number of individuals or are you more concerned about the privacy of the information and limiting access to it?

For many family caregivers, the best place to start is with paper. A simple pocket folder or three-ring binder is the perfect place to store hard copies of the documents you collect. The folder or binder can be easily stored and taken with you when going to see a healthcare provider. Organizing physicians' records by date, with the most recent doctors' notes in the front, will make life easier should you need to access this information quickly.

If you are more computer-savvy and you believe that your loved one's healthcare providers are as well, then you may decide to store the PHR on a floppy disk or a portable device like a memory stick that can easily be carried with you from one provider to the next. While even less cumbersome to carry than a file folder or binder, this type of storage method only works if the people who will most likely be accessing the information have the technology that will allow them to retrieve it when they need it.

If you are concerned about the ability to access your loved one's information anywhere at any time without having to remember to carry that information on your person, then you may want to evaluate the various Web-based options available. A number of companies will provide you with a private online account that can be accessed by anyone you give permission to at any time, day or night. A few of these services will even collect and organize health records for you, a feature that is particularly helpful if your loved one sees multiple physicians and/or you don't want the burden of data collection yourself. Many of these companies will store the information on a CD for you, and will fax or mail the information as needed. These Web-based services may be the best answer for you if you are concerned about finding yourself in an emergency situation or if you and your loved one are often away from home. Do find out about each particular vendor's security system, however, as privacy and confidentiality of information should be an important consideration when choosing a company to use. Make sure the PHR will be securely stored, and that the only people who will be able to access the information will be the ones you and your care recipient designate. Prices for these Web-based companies vary, as do the exact services they provide, so do your homework carefully and ask questions before choosing a service.

The American Health Information Management Association maintains a list of PHR service providers on its consumer-focused Web site, www.myphr.com. You can link to companies that specialize in the offline storage of records (e.g., a self-contained binder or CD-ROM) as well as companies that will maintain these records for you electronically via the Internet. You can even view a list of companies that provide PHR tools for free.

Whichever format you choose to collect and store health information, the important thing is that you do make a choice.

While the reality of your life as a family caregiver may make this undertaking seem impossible, remember that not all the pieces need to come together at once, and you don't have to be the one organizing it all. This would be a great project to farm out to a willing family member or friend. The important thing is to begin the process, slowly if necessary. If the prospect of gathering all of the information listed above is too overwhelming, start with the information you think is most important. Here's how to get started:

- Label a file folder or binder in which you will store this information and designate a spot in your home where this folder or binder will be kept so that it is easily accessible, especially in the case of an emergency.
- Create a simple document with basic information to form the core of the record: your loved one's name, address, and phone number. List all of his or her doctors and their contact information and the medications being taken, including dosage instructions. List all relevant medical conditions and functional issues (e.g., uses a wheelchair, has poor short-term memory). Don't forget to put in your name and contact information as the primary family caregiver.
- Identify the healthcare providers from whom you need to collect medical records.
- Fill out the appropriate authorization forms. These forms, as well as many other tools you need to get started, are available on a number of Web sites, many of which can be accessed by going to www.myphr.com. Even the services that charge monthly or annual fees often make certain PHR tools available for free through their Web sites. Explore these sites and evaluate what the various companies have to offer, and what these services will cost you.
- Finally, as you begin the process of creating a PHR for your loved one, *don't forget to create a PHR for another very important person: YOU!*

The American Health Information Management Association (AHIMA) has created a free public Web site where you can find a wide range of helpful information, resources, and a searchable database of PHR products and services. You can take advantage of a wealth of information and advice from a source you can trust. Go to www.myphr.com.

—Sandy Padwo Rogers is the managing editor of TAKE CARE!

Making the Most of the Doctor's Office Visit

The following information is excerpted from the take-home guide of the "Communicating Effectively with Healthcare Professionals" workshop, developed by NFCA. The workshop provides family caregivers with the practical information needed to communicate well in healthcare settings.

Visiting the doctor's office with your loved one can be a stressful experience, for both of you. The time you have with the doctor is extremely short and goes by unbelievably quickly. No doubt you will have many questions and concerns that you would like addressed during this time. How can you ensure that you get the most out of each and every doctor's visit? Whether the appointment is for a regular checkup or the result of an acute illness or injury, investing a little time and effort prior to the visit will help ensure that both you and your loved one are satisfied at its conclusion.

Learn How the Doctor's Office Functions
You have probably noticed that doctors' offices seem to have personalities, just like people. It depends partly on size, type, and location of the practice. (You won't have the same experience with a twelve-physician surgical-group practice in a Chicago skyscraper that you will have with a solo pediatrician in a rural Minnesota clinic.) Despite all the variation, there are some things that doctors' offices have in common. By learning how their office systems work, you and your loved one have a better chance for a positive healthcare experience.

Find Out Who Can Answer Your Questions
Usually, doctors do not have time to answer questions over the phone. Most offices prefer that you start by talking with a nurse or a physician's assistant. These healthcare professionals may be able to:

- Make appointments
- Answer general medical questions
- Look up information in your care recipient's chart

- Provide test results
- Confirm correct medications and dosages
- Help arrange for prescription refills, etc.
- Help with medical emergencies

They also can consult with the doctor between patients and get back to you relatively quickly with answers to your questions. If you have complicated questions, however, don't be afraid to ask to speak with the doctor. The staff will help you determine who can best address your concerns. Learning the names of the office staff can go a long way in helping you establish personal and cooperative relationships.

Determine the Best Time to Reach the Doctor

Some doctors have specific hours during which they take calls or answer faxes and e-mail messages. If your physician is one of these, find out when this is and call during that time. If the doctor you are working with does not have specific "call-back" hours, leave a message with the receptionist in the morning. It will speed things up if the doctor has some idea of why you're calling, so give the receptionist a one-sentence summary of your primary question. Also, leave all of the numbers where you can be reached at various times during the day.

Learn How to Deal with Medical Emergencies

Most doctors suggest that you go to the ER if you have an emergency after office hours. Ask your doctor if he or she has specific instructions or if you should bring your loved one to the office during business hours. It's helpful to get answers to the following questions:

- Who should you call after hours or when the doctor isn't available?
- How should medical emergencies be handled?
- Which emergency facility does the doctor prefer you to use?

- At which hospitals and specialty clinics does the doctor have practice privileges?
- If the doctor does not have privileges at the nearest hospital to you, what does he or she recommend in the case of an emergency?

Prepare for the Office Visit

Most people wouldn't dream of going to the grocery store without some idea of what they want to purchase. They check their cupboards and refrigerator and take stock of what they need. While taking your loved one to the doctor is definitely not the same as grocery shopping, it also requires taking stock—of your loved one's current health status and the reasons for the office visit.

Before the Visit

Establish/Check the Patient File

The single most important thing you can do to promote clear communication and function effectively as a family caregiver is to create and maintain a comprehensive file of information about your loved one. All of your questions, notes, medical records, and instructions from healthcare professionals should go in this notebook.

When you are preparing for any healthcare encounter, you should plan to take this file with you. Before the office visit, quickly skim through the file to make sure it's up-to-date. If your loved one sees more than one physician, be sure that your file includes the latest physician notes or any hospital discharge papers that you have received. You may want to make copies of the pages that have important information so that you can simply give the doctor a copy.

Gather Your Questions

Before you and your loved one visit any healthcare provider, write down the questions you have for the doctor. You may want to write these questions in your loved one's notebook/file so that you have everything in one place when you go for the office visit.

Identify Current Symptoms

Think through your loved one's current condition before the office visit. Make a list that includes the current state of and any changes in your loved one's overall wellbeing. This list should include information on his general condition, including any changes in pain, medications, and emotional and mental wellbeing. If possible, share your observations with your care recipient. Ideally, you will both "be on the same page" in terms of what you are observing. If not, you may need to find a way to convey your thoughts directly to the doctor so that he or she has a clear picture about your loved one's situation. (See "Help with Reporting" below.)

Call to Confirm the Appointment

Scheduling mistakes happen. Physicians have emergencies. Because a trip to the doctor may be a physically challenging endeavor, and because you may be taking valuable time from work or another equally important activity, it's wise to call the doctor's office the day of the appointment. Call a couple of hours before your scheduled visit, or just before you are getting ready to leave, to make sure the doctor is on schedule and no last-minute emergencies have popped up.

Don't Forget to Ask About Billing Practices

If your loved one is seeing a new physician for the first time, it's a good idea to find out as much as you can about the doctor's billing practices. Some questions to keep in mind:

- Does the office accept your care recipient's health insurance?
- Who is responsible for filing insurance claims?
- What are the charges for typical services, such as a standard office visit?
- What forms of payment does the office accept in addition to cash? Personal checks? Credit cards?
- If your loved one is eligible for Medicaid and/or

Medicare, does the office accept those as full payment for care, or is there an additional charge?

- Who is the best person to talk with about billing and insurance questions?
- What forms need to be signed so that the doctor's office can give treatment, bill the insurance company, and provide other services?

During the Visit

Help with Reporting

The office visit is for the patient, of course, not for you. Your care recipient should take the lead, if possible. If you are in the doctor's office during the consultation, listen carefully to what everyone says. If necessary, help fill in the gaps in your loved one's reporting and gently correct anything you believe to be wrong or incomplete. Legally, the doctor isn't even supposed to talk to the family caregiver because of privacy regulations. Hopefully, your loved one's doctor doesn't stand on principle, but, rather, compassion and common sense. However, just to make sure you don't run into problems participating in the visit if you want to, your loved one should tell the doctor (if possible) that he or she wants you to be present. It's best to put this in writing.

Describe Symptoms Accurately

It is best to start with what you think are the most significant changes and symptoms. Always be as clear and thorough as you can when reporting symptoms; details are critical when it comes to diagnoses and treatments.

Ask Questions

Go through the questions you wrote in your notebook and discuss them briefly with the doctor. Then write down the answers. If you don't understand something that comes up in the conversation, ask questions, and tell the doctor you need information clarified if you are to do your job as the family caregiver.

Record the Doctor's Instructions

Take notes about any changes the doctor suggests in treatments, home care, medications, and other things related to your loved one's care. These notes don't have to be extensive—just enough to help you remember clearly what needs to be done and why.

Discuss Recommendations

Make sure you understand the reasons for—and results expected from—any recommended medical tests, surgical procedures, or new therapies. Ask questions until you thoroughly understand what is going to happen and why. Have the doctor describe the potential side effects of a new medication or treatment. Don't leave the office visit until you understand.

Verify Follow-Up

As the visit winds down, ask when you should call the office to get any test results. If the doctor does not tell you when the next appointment should take place, ask when it should be and what to expect next.

After the Visit

Review Your Notes

Look at your notes. Is there anything you don't understand now that you're home? If so, call the office within twenty-four hours to clarify things.

Check Prescriptions

Double-check that any prescriptions were filled correctly at the pharmacy. For more on this subject, see page 212.

Discuss the Visit

Ask your loved one how he feels about the office visit and what he learned. Discuss anything that will need to be handled differently as a result of the visit.

Update Your Calendar

    Put the date of the next visit in your calendar right away.

Call for Test Results

    Call about test results on the day the doctor's office indicated they would be available. Get copies for your file. If you don't understand something on the report, don't hesitate to have someone in the doctor's office explain it to you. Understanding test results when you first get them can sometimes prevent significant problems down the road.

    As your loved one's care coordinator, you wear a variety of hats. When it comes to the doctor's office visit, you serve as your loved one's voice when needed, you advocate on his behalf, and you are the one to whom the physician turns to ensure that the treatment plan is followed.

    You can help facilitate a productive and satisfying healthcare encounter by coming armed with the information the physician needs, by helping your loved one communicate clearly, by actively listening, and by ensuring that your loved one complies with the treatment plan. As part of the healthcare team, you can help make the most out of the visit to the physician's office.

Improving Doctor–Caregiver Communications

There is much to be gained by improving communications between family caregivers and healthcare professionals, especially physicians. Positive outcomes include: better care for the patient, less stress and illness on the part of the caregiver, more efficient use of doctors' time, reduced costs, and more satisfaction for all concerned.

    In order to reap these benefits caregivers and physicians need to gain a better understanding of each other's worlds. They need to try, as hard as it is, to "walk in each other's shoes."

    The following guide is offered as a path for doing just that.

Tips for Doctors from Family Caregivers

- Be open and forthright.
- Think about the practicality of the treatments you suggest and consider their effect on the entire family, not just their medical efficacy.
- When you prescribe medications, be sure caregivers understand potential side effects so they know what to expect.
- In non-life-threatening situations, assure caregivers that every decision doesn't have to be made on the spot. Respect the right of the caregiver and the patient to think things over.
- Now and then ask the caregiver, "How are you?" Let them know you understand that illness and disability are family affairs.
- Be accessible, especially when a caregiver is opening his or her heart.
- Reach out to the caregiver, literally. A simple touch can mean a great deal.
- Be sensitive about where you talk to caregivers about difficult subjects—waiting rooms and corridors are not appropriate.
- Always explain as completely as possible all of the legal ramifications of life-saving actions.
- Be prepared to tell caregivers about helpful resources. Living with a chronic illness or disability requires more than medicine has to offer.

Tips for Family Caregivers from Physicians and Other Healthcare Professionals

- Write questions down so you won't forget them.
- Be clear about what you want to say to the doctor. Try not to ramble.
- If you have many things to talk about, make a consultation appointment so the doctor can allow enough

time to meet with you in an unhurried way.

- Educate yourself about your loved one's disease or disability. With all the information on the Internet it is easier than ever before.

- Learn the routine at your doctor's office and/or the hospital so you can make the system work for you, not against you.

- Recognize that not all questions have answers—especially those beginning with "why."

- Separate your anger and sense of impotence about not being able to help your loved one as much as you would like from your feelings about the doctor. Remember, you are both on the same side.

- Appreciate what the doctor is doing to help and say thank you from time to time.

Preventing Medication Mishaps

As family caregivers we play a significant role in ensuring our loved ones' safety as they interact with healthcare providers. We monitor their wellbeing and report symptoms. We advocate for their rights to treatment, and we manage their medications. And there are so many medications!

Chronically ill or disabled individuals take more medications than any other group of individuals. They see more doctors as well, each one focused on a different condition. Unfortunately, our loved ones' doctors don't usually talk to each other, so they are unfamiliar with the full list of drugs that have been prescribed. That being the case, it isn't surprising that adverse events from medication interactions are the leading cause of visits to the ER. That's scary news, but there are some fairly easy things that you can do to prevent medication mishaps.

- First and foremost, maintain an up-to-date list of everything your loved one takes. List medications prescribed by doctors, but also list those purchased without a prescription, such as aspirin, vitamins, and herbal supplements. These over-the-counter "meds" can, at times, interact with prescription drugs and create serious problems. You are probably the only one who knows all the medications your loved one is taking, especially if he or she sees multiple physicians.

  Be sure to list the name, dosage, and frequency of the medication (e.g., Warfarin, four mg, once a day), the reason for taking it, (blood-clot prevention), any dosing directions (may be taken with or without food), and the start date. For prescription drugs add the name and number of the prescribing doctor, and the name and number of the pharmacy that filled the prescription.

  Be sure to put your loved one's name at the top of the document and include your contact information (or someone else's) as the person to call in an emergency.

  Note any allergies or intolerances, or other significant medical information that might not be obvious.

Make multiple copies, one for you to carry and one for your loved one's personal medical file. Keep one on the refrigerator for paramedics to find, and send a copy to your loved one's primary doctor.

It is critical that you keep this record updated. Not only will an outdated record not do any good, but it may actually do harm. A simple computer-based document you create yourself is one of the easiest ways to keep the record current.

- We all know that doctors are notorious for having bad handwriting. Don't be shy about asking all your loved one's doctors to "translate" their handwriting so you can write down exactly what a prescribed medication is, its name, dosage, etc.

- On each medicine bottle, write down the name of the condition it treats. You might find that your loved one is taking three different pills for the same condition, each prescribed by a different physician. That may be exactly what is needed, but it is definitely a red flag to alert you to ask questions.

- Try to use the same pharmacy for all prescriptions. That way there will be an official record of all your loved one's prescription medications over an extended period of time.

- When your loved one is prescribed a new medication, ask the doctor and pharmacist about potential side effects and interactions with others drugs, vitamins, or foods. But don't stop there. You can check for side effects and interactions yourself online. If you get conflicting information, start asking questions. Monitor your loved one for reactions and, at the first sign of trouble, call the doctor and report the specific symptoms you see.

With the aging of the population, healthier living conditions, and the fruits of scientific research allowing all of us to live longer, our use of prescription medications is only going to increase. Following these simple rules can help you prevent problems caused by interactions between medications, vitamins, supplements, and foods. It is one more way that you can be a good steward of your loved one's health. It is also a good example of what it means to be a proactive family caregiver. And while you are following these steps to protect your loved one's health, consider following them for yourself as well. Remember, your own good health is essential to your wellbeing and your ability to be an effective family caregiver.

APPENDIX D

Finances

Tax Tips for Family Caregivers
by Cecily Slater, CPA

Do you dread April 15? Family caregivers in particular have good reason to feel stressed about this day. The role of family caregiver, by its very nature, is one that often places you in a challenging financial position. There may be one bright spot to April 15, however. As a family caregiver, you may be entitled to deductions or credits that can help take some of the sting out of tax season. The following tips should serve as a guide for you to begin thinking about how to maximize your deductions. Tax rules change, so always check with a tax professional when you are getting ready to file.

Medical Expense Deductions: General Principles

For a deduction to qualify as a medical expense, you must have spent money to alleviate or prevent a physical or mental defect or illness. Common deductions include:

- Medical insurance premiums (unless pretax)
- Prescription medicines
- Doctors' bills

215

- Hospital fees for services and/or room and board
- Travel to and from medical appointments (The mileage rate for 2006 is eighteen cents per mile.)

You can deduct only medical and dental expenses that are in excess of 7.5 percent of your adjusted gross income (AGI). For example, if your AGI is $25,000 and your medical expenses add up to $2,000, you will be able to deduct only $125. That's the difference between the $2,000 you spent and $1,875, which is 7.5 percent of $25,000. There's another catch: You can deduct only those amounts for which you have not been reimbursed by private insurance or Medicare. If you are in the upper tax brackets, some itemized deductions are phased out altogether. Deductible medical expenses are *not* subject to this reduction, however.

Special Expenses

You can claim the following special items as medical deductions:

- Oxygen and oxygen equipment
- Special schools or homes for the mentally or physically disabled (when recommended by a doctor)
- Artificial limbs
- False teeth
- Eyeglasses
- Wheelchairs and repairs
- Crutches
- Costs and care of guide dogs for aiding the disabled
- Braille books and magazines if they are more expensive than regular books and magazines
- Hearing aids and the batteries to operate them
- Travel costs including lodging to receive medical treatment

You can also deduct expenses for equipment or improvements you've made to your home for medical reasons, but the

IRS will reduce these deductions by the amount such improvements increase the value of your home. Typical equipment and improvements added initially for medical reasons include:

- Ramps
- Widened doorways and hallways
- Grab bars in bathrooms
- Elevators, stair glides, etc.
- Air conditioning
- Accessible shower stalls

Unfortunately, health-club dues and dancing or swimming lessons are not deductible, even if recommended by a doctor.

Nursing Home Care

Nursing home expenses, per se, are not deductible, but medical expenses incurred in a nursing home are. This includes the cost of meals and lodging while the patient is in the nursing home, so long as the main reason for being there is to get medical (not simply personal) care.

Nursing, Therapeutic, and/or Aide Services

Wages you pay for an attendant who provides nursing and/or personal care services are deductible as medical expenses. These services include such nursing activities as giving medication and changing dressings, and typical personal care services such as bathing and grooming the patient. If you provide room and board, these may also be deductible, but typical household services such as cooking and cleaning do not qualify as medical deductions.

For Whom Can You Claim Medical Deductions?

You can take medical-expense deductions for yourself, your spouse, and your dependents. A person generally qualifies as a dependent for medical expense deductions if he or she meets all of the following criteria:

- Is related to you
- Lived with you for the entire year as a member of your household (Parents, children over the age of nineteen, grandchildren, and siblings do not have to meet this requirement.)
- Was a U.S. citizen or resident, or a resident of Canada or Mexico, for at least part of the calendar year for which you are filing taxes
- You provided over half of that person's total support for the calendar year. If you and someone else are providing more than half a dependent's support, but no one alone provides more than half, you can use what's called a "multiple support agreement" to claim the dependent, but only one of the parties to the agreement can claim medical expenses for the dependent person. (For example, to take the medical deduction for expenses of a parent, the adult child must be providing 50 percent or more of the support for the parent. If several siblings combined contribute 50 percent, but no single child pays the 50 percent, a multiple support agreement can be filed with the return and one of the siblings may claim the expenses.) If parents of a child with significant medical expenses are divorced parents, the child is considered a dependent of both parents for the medical-expense deduction.

Where to Get Help

Tax law is confusing at best. If you want some additional information, here are ways to get it:

- The Internal Revenue Service offers a number of publications that can help you understand the deductions and tax credits to which you may be entitled. Some of the most helpful include:
  - ° Your Federal Income Tax: Publication 17
  - ° Medical and Dental Expenses: Publication 502
  - ° Credit for the Elderly or Disabled: Publication 554

°   Tax Rules for Children and Dependents: Publication 929. To order these publications, call 800-TAX-FORM.

- The IRS will also answer taxpayer questions if they are not too complicated or controversial. You must realize, however, that while the IRS will try to guide you in finding the answers you need, it does not offer tax advice. To find the Taxpayer Service Number for your area, check the local phone book under the IRS listings.

- There is only one place to go for individual tax advice, and that is to a tax professional. If you are confused about what deductions or credits may apply to you, or if you need help preparing your return, you may find it beneficial to consult someone who specializes in this area. There are a number of tax services available, and you can find their numbers in the phone book, but the best reference may well be word of mouth. Talk to people you know and respect and ask them for a referral.

—Cecily Slater is a certified public accountant who has been providing tax and financial planning advice to individuals and businesses in the greater Washington, DC, area since 1979.

Financial Management:
A Guide for Family Caregivers
by Paula McCarron

Have you ever calculated the cost of caring? Certainly as a family caregiver, your service to your loved one is beyond measure in terms of the love, depth of care, and concern you offer. If you were to take a look at some of the "real" dollar costs of caring, however, here's what you would learn:

- In 2000, the family caregivers who stopped working to provide full-time care lost approximately $109 per day in wages and health benefits.[1]
- The value of "free care" provided by family caregivers is estimated to be $306 billion a year. That is virtually twice the amount actually spent on home-care and nursing-home services by the government or private insurance combined.[2]
- Insurance experts estimate that about one-third of all long-term care services are paid for by individuals out of their own savings or investments.[3]
- The national average wage for a health aide is $18 an hour[4] and the average cost of a one-month stay in an assisted living home is $2,524.[5]

Confronted with facts like these, it's clear that being a family caregiver without a financial plan is risky business—for both you and your loved one.

Whether you are providing care for a child, spouse, or parent, you are your care recipient's most important asset. That's why it's necessary that a financial plan be put in place in case you can no longer continue providing care, either temporarily or permanently.

With that in mind, every family caregiver should consider two crucial questions:

1. How can you ensure that your loved one's needs are met if you become disabled or ill, or if you die?

2. What kinds of financial protections and insurance can you put into place now to protect yourself and your loved one down the road?

Know Your Options

"It's important to know your options, whether or not you choose to use them," says Jay Bell, vice president of education with the National Endowment for Financial Education. To know your options, you first need to know your assets. Assets typically include: earnings, pension funds, Social Security benefits, property such as homes or land, insurance, retirement funds, and so on.

Mark Darrell, CFP, of Darrell Financial, a financial planning firm based in Baltimore, Maryland, agrees. The process of financial planning, Darrell explains, involves a review of one's assets, discussion of options, creation of a plan for the future, and education on the kinds and amounts of insurance that may be needed to ensure that future. "Eighty percent of families are living paycheck to paycheck," says Darrell. "They tell me they can't afford to go on vacation much less spend money on insurance. But even if they can't do everything, they can often do something. And it's better to have something in the event you need it than to end up with nothing."

When it comes to replacing the long-term care services you provide your loved one (or planning on how to cover your own needs in the future), Darrell notes there are four basic avenues to pursue:

1. Use your savings.
2. Convert an asset into cash.
3. Obtain assistance from family.
4. Make use of insurance.

Start Saving Today

Family caregivers assume that nothing is going to happen to them; unfortunately, that isn't always true. If something does happen, you need to be prepared. Funding a replacement for *you* could be an expensive proposition. The most important step you can take now is to create a savings plan that you can draw from quickly in the event of an emergency. But don't stop there. Start saving today to ensure that you have adequate income for your retirement. To build retirement savings, you might consider setting up an IRA or contributing to a 401(k) plan through your employer. Many employers will match employee contributions to a 401(k) plan, either dollar-for-dollar or with some percentage of each dollar saved. Both IRAs and 401(k) plans allow you to build for the future while enjoying some tax savings now. No matter how much or how little you have to contribute, the key is to begin to save something today. IRAs and 401(k) plans can be tapped in an emergency, although this may not be the best option because of possible tax consequences. As noted above, it is better to have more liquid savings available.

Converting Assets into Cash

The quickest way to convert assets into cash is to sell something that is relatively liquid: stock or mutual funds, for example. Less liquid financial assets include CDs, IRAs, 401(k) plans, or other retirement accounts. Before you sell any financial asset, it's important to look at the big picture. There may be penalties for early withdrawals, or taxes to pay, all of which mean you could actually lose money. So look before you leap and understand all of the ramifications of your decision.

The biggest asset most of us have is our home; there are a number of ways to convert some of its value into cash. Home equity loans let you write checks whenever you want based on a preapproved line of credit that is tied to the amount of equity you have accrued in your home. Once established, a home equity loan makes the money readily available. This is a loan, however, and the money must be repaid, with interest.

A relatively new way to convert your home's equity into cash is the reverse mortgage. It provides tax-free income to eligible individuals 62 years of age or older and allows homeowners to stay in their homes as long as they like, without adding new mortgage payments.

"The reverse mortgage is aptly named because the payment stream is 'reversed.' Instead of making monthly payments to a lender, as with a regular mortgage, a lender makes payments to you," says Peter Bell, executive director of the National Reverse Mortgage Lenders Association. Reverse mortgages are complicated; anyone who is considering one must first meet with an approved counselor to ensure they understand all of the ramifications of this type of mortgage. The counselor's job is to educate you about reverse mortgages, to inform you of other options available, and to assist you in determining which particular reverse mortgage product best fits your needs.

Protect Your Income in the Event of Disability

If you are in the workforce, disability insurance is one level of protection that can keep income flowing if you are unable to work due to illness, injury, or disability. While there is no disability insurance that will cover 100 percent of your income, you may be able to secure enough coverage to replace 60 percent to 80 percent of your income.

Disability insurance is often offered by employers at very minimal cost, and can also be purchased privately. It may be available as a rider on an existing life insurance plan or through a group or professional association. You can also purchase an individual plan from an insurance broker or get competitive quotes by shopping for rates online. No matter what you choose to do, be sure to check with your state's insurance commissioner's office to find out if the agent and company are licensed to operate in your state.

Some people may think they will qualify for disability benefits under Social Security; however, Social Security disability is very limited, as it does not allow for "partial" or "temporary" disability. In addition to restrictive eligibility criteria, it can take up to five months to qualify for benefits and up to two years to process claims.

When purchasing disability insurance, be sure to ask these questions:

- What is the company's definition of disability?
- Who makes the determination of disability?
- When do benefits begin?
- What percentage of income would be replaced and for how long?
- Does the plan factor for inflation?
- Does the plan cover only illness or accident, or both?
- Can the policy be renewed? Is there a clause addressing non-cancellation?

Disability insurance premiums vary greatly depending on your occupation, age, income, elimination periods, and so on. As with any insurance product, it is best to shop around.

Don't Overlook the Importance of Life Insurance

If you don't already have a life insurance policy in place, consider the following questions:

- If you die, who is going to fill your shoes as a family caregiver so that your loved one continues to receive the care that he or she needs?
- Where will the money come from to provide the services that you have been providing for "free"?

For many family caregivers, a life insurance policy can offer peace of mind that their loved ones' needs, as well as their own future care needs, will be met.

"There's no rule of thumb about what kind of policy to buy or in what amounts," says Darrell. "You've got to consider every situation independently on its own terms. That's why I suggest that people seek the help of a broker who can represent many companies and many plans instead of an agent who works only for one company."

Just like agents who represent only one company, brokers are paid through a built-in fee whenever an insurance plan is sold. Unlike agents, brokers do not represent any one company and, therefore, can show you a variety of plans from several companies. To find a broker, contact your state's insurance commissioner's office or get referrals from trusted family members or friends.

How can life insurance help you meet your long-term care needs? First, family caregivers can purchase life insurance to ensure an adequate income for their care recipients or to help cover the costs of obtaining long-term care services if the family caregiver should die. Second, there are ways for care recipients to make use of their own life insurance policies to fund their long-term care costs. A care recipient may be eligible to make a tax-free cash withdrawal to fund long-term care expenses under some policies. Any remaining funds are paid to heirs when the policyholder dies.

Another option is to obtain a viatical settlement. This is more commonly used for an individual who has a limited life expectancy. Here's how it works: Mary names the viatical company as the sole beneficiary of her life insurance policy and, in return, she receives an immediate cash payout of up to 85 percent of the policy's face value. When Mary dies, the viatical company will receive the policy's death benefit.

"Before anyone opts for any of these kinds of settlements, it's important to know the possible penalties involved and the tax consequences," says Darrell. "That's why every decision must be made with the view of the whole financial picture." In fact, according to Darrell, any time you move money around or cash out an investment, it's important to look at the whole picture. "Otherwise," he says, "you might actually end up losing money."

Consider Buying Long-Term Care Insurance

Whereas disability insurance can replace some of your income if you are laid up for a time, long-term care insurance can cover the costs of your own care needs. Long-term care insurance is not for everyone, though. "It's really designed for people who have the desire and need to protect assets," says Keith Eig, of Greenberg, Wexler and Eig, an insurance consulting business in Maryland. Family caregivers may want to consider this type of insurance as a way to maintain control over how and where care is received in the future. Because of the variations in benefits and types of coverage, however, long-term care insurance is both complicated and expensive, notes Eig. "You want to be sure to choose a company that is making you a promise it can live up to," says Eig. "That means you need to shop carefully."

Some long-term care policies will provide a set level of reimbursement for each day, whether or not you actually spend the money on needed services; other plans will provide reimbursement for actual dollars spent. Some plans offer fixed periods of benefit duration while others offer lifetime coverage.

Long-term care insurance typically covers services such as home-health aides, adult day services, assisted-living homes, and nursing-home care. However, some policies may cover only services provided by a registered nurse or a certified home-health aide while others may allow for the hire of a family member or friend. In some situations, the insurance company will arrange for a care manager who will preapprove all services. Under other policies, an individual may receive a fixed "payout"—for example, $200 a day—that may be used in any way that the individual chooses. It's important to know the maximum benefit limit of the policy as well as the duration of the coverage period.

The Bottom Line

Ensuring a financially healthy future for you and your loved one will take research, analysis, and the willingness to make some difficult decisions. It's not necessary to do everything today; but it *is* necessary to begin to take the steps that will help you and your loved one be better prepared for whatever the future holds. As a family caregiver, you know better than anyone that the next health crisis is not a matter of "if," but "when." Laying the groundwork today will help you ensure that your financial needs—and those of your loved one—are met tomorrow.

Choosing a Financial Planner

Most certified financial planners offer a free initial consultation. "That way the planner can learn a bit more about your situation and you can determine if you feel comfortable with the planner," says Mark Darrell. Use that time to ask about fees, types of services provided, and what kinds of reports you will receive. Know if you are paying for services based on hourly rates or if there are any additional costs or fees.

No matter what kind of financial planner you choose to hire, it's critical to check on his or her background. Asking friends or attorneys for referrals can be one way to find a good financial planner. Ask about credentials, education, and experience to be sure you are hiring a planner who understands your particular needs.

Resources

1. Joy Loverde, *The Complete Eldercare Planner*, 2nd ed. (Three Rivers Press, 2000).

2. Eric Tyson, MBA, *Personal Finance for Dummies*, 4th ed. (Wiley Publishing, Inc., 2003).

3. "With Open Arms: Embracing a Bright Financial Future for You and Your Child"

    A seventy-two-page financial guide for adults caring for children with disabilities or other special needs. The booklet is available as a free download from www.easterseals.com or for purchase ($5) by phoning 800-221-6827.

4. National Association of Insurance Commissioners (NAIC)
    816-783-8300
    www.naic.org

    NAIC will help you locate your state's insurance commissioner's office. NAIC also offers consumer guides on the purchase of life insurance, long-term care insurance, and other types of insurance. Check out the NAIC publication "A Shopper's Guide to Long-Term Care Insurance." It can be obtained through the NAIC Web site.

5. National Endowment for Financial Education
www.nefe.org
Many informative and "reader-friendly" articles are available on this Web site.

—Paula McCarron is a freelance health writer living in Massachusetts. She has been involved in nursing home, hospice, and home-based care for more than twenty years.

Endnotes

1. B. R. Stucki and J. Mulvey, "Can Aging Baby Boomers Avoid the Nursing Home? Long-Term Care Insurance for 'Aging in Place'" (American Council of Life Insurers, March 2000).
2. Peter S. Arno, "Economic Value of Informal Caregiving," presented at the Care Coordination and the Caregiver Forum of the Department of Veterans Affairs, National Institutes of Health, Bethesda, MD January 25–27, 2006.
3. Testimony of Buck Stinson, president of Long-Term Care Division, Government Relations, Genworth Financial, before the Subcommittee on Health of the House Committee on Ways and Means, April 19, 2005.
4. MetLife Mature Market Institute, 2004 MetLife Market Survey of Nursing Home and Home Care Costs, September 27, 2004, Press Release, www.metlife.com.
5. MetLife Mature Market Institute, 2004 MetLife Market Survey of Assisted Living Costs, October 25, 2004, Press Release, www.metlife.com.

Selective Chapter Bibliography

Only books, articles, and studies specifically mentioned by name in the text are included here. Many more sources were used in researching information for this book.

Introduction
Levine Carol, ed. *Always on Call: When Illness Turns Families into Caregivers*. New York: United Hospital Fund (2000) 2.

Chapter 1
Styron, William. *Darkness Visible: A Memoir of Madness*. New York: Random House, (1990), 50.

Chapter 2
Cassidy Wiggins, Rita. *Shedding Light: Poems About Living with Alzheimer's*. St. Helena: Ten Press, (2000) 13.

Dickinson, Peter. *Some Death before Dying*. New York: Mysterious Press, Warner Books, (1999) 21.

Mace, Nancy L., MA; and Rabins, Peter V., M.D., M. P.H. *36 Hour Day: A Family Guide to Caring for Someone with Alzheimer's Disease, Related Dementing Illnesses, and Memory Loss in Later Life*. Baltimore: Johns Hopkins Press, 1999.

Chapter 3
Casarett, DJ; Karlawish, JH; Byock, I. "Advocacy and activism: missing pieces in the quest to improve end-of-life care." J Palliat Med. Feb 2002;5(1):3-12.

"Disability and American Families: 2000," *Census 2000 Special Reports*, July 2005.

"Evercare Study of Caregivers in Decline" (Press Release). Evercare and National Alliance for Caregiving, September 2006.

Institute of Medicine, *To Err Is Human: Building a Safer Health System*, National Academy Press, Washington, DC (2000).

Lazaroff, Alan MD. Testimony "Cash Crunch: The Financial Challenge of LTC" Washington: Senate Special Committee on Aging (March 9, 1998).

Levine, Carol *Rough Crossings: Family Caregivers' Odysseys through the Health Care System*. New York: United Hospital Fund, (2000) 9, 11-13.

Mintz, Suzanne. Testimony "Who Cares for the Caregivers: The Role of Health Insurance in Promoting Quality Care for Seniors, Children, and Individuals with Disabilities." Senate Subcommittee on Oversight of Government Management Restructuring Washington, DC (July 24, 2000).

National Family Caregivers Association, Survey of Self-Identified Family Caregivers, 2001.

Shellenbarger, Sue "Work & Family" *Wall Street Journal*, 13 September, 2000.

Chapter 5

Bly, Robert, *Morning Poems*. New York: Harper Collins (1997).

Clooney, Eleanor "Death in Slow Motion: A Descent into Alzheimer's," *Harper's Magazine*, Vol 303 # 19817 (2001): 43 –58.

Jivanjee, Pauline, PhD; Simpson, Jennifer PhD, "Respite Care for Children with Serious Emotional Disorders and Their Families: A Way to Enrich Family Life." *Focal Point*, Regional Research Institute for Human Services, Portland State University, Vol 15 No 2 (2001).

About the Author

Suzanne Geffen Mintz, President/Co-founder
National Family Caregivers Association

Suzanne Mintz is a social entrepreneur. She took a personal experience, her husband's diagnosis of MS and its ensuing impact on their lives, and built a national organization to improve the lives of family caregivers, the National Family Caregivers Association (NFCA). She has transformed the lens through which healthcare professionals, public policy makers, the media, and the general public view family caregiving and has empowered hundreds of thousands of individual family caregivers to take charge of their own lives and speak up on behalf of themselves and their loved ones.

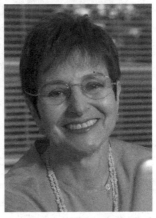

Photo by D. Peck

Ms. Mintz is currently president of the organization she co-founded almost fifteen years ago as the only national organization for all family caregivers, regardless of their loved one's age or diagnosis. She recognized early in this journey that the impact of family caregiving goes beyond individual families and has become a national healthcare and social policy issue. Suzanne has testified before Congress and is often quoted by the national press.

In 2006 she was one of fifteen winners, out of an initial

pool of 1,200, for the first-ever Purpose Prize, a national award for Americans sixty and above who are leading a new age of social innovation. Suzanne is also the 2004 recipient of the Lifetime Achievement Award from the Eli Lilly Welcome Back initiative.

Besides *A Family Caregiver Speaks Up* (the updated and revised edition of *Love, Honor & Value*), Suzanne Mintz is the author of *The Resourceful Caregiver* and numerous articles and educational pamphlets.

Ms. Mintz is a member of the board of the National Health Council, the Board of Governors of the National Patient Safety Foundation, and the Advisory Board of the Partnership to Fight Chronic Disease.

Suzanne holds a bachelors degree in English from Queens College University of the City of New York and a master's degree in human ecology from the University of Maryland.

She lives in Kensington, Maryland, with her husband Steven and their cat KC.

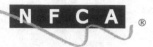

NATIONAL FAMILY CAREGIVERS ASSOCIATION

An Invitation for Family Caregivers
Become part of NFCA's *Family Caregiver Community!*

Access the latest resources, connect with others, and find support with NFCA's Family Caregiver Community . . .

Throughout the year, we offer family caregivers who sign up FREE resources like:

- An online story bank with stories from caregivers across the country
- A Pen Pal program that connects you directly with others who are caring for loved ones
- An educational library with resources to support your day-to-day responsibilities
- NFCA's popular newsletter, called *TAKE CARE!*, with information and resources about the experiences of caregiving.

Becoming part of *NFCA's Family Caregiver Community* is easy and free. Sign up today by visiting www.thefamilycaregiver.org and click on the "Family Caregiver Sign Up" button or call 1-800-896-3650.

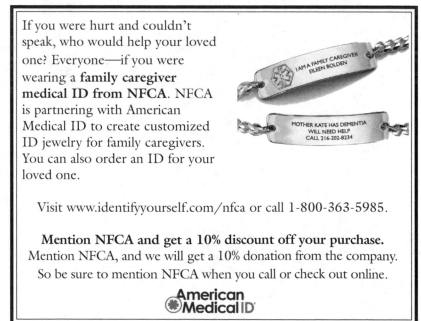